Laparoscopic hysterectomy and oophorectomy:

A practical manual and colour atlas

For Churchill Livingstone

Publisher: Peter Richardson
Copy Editor: Susan Hunter
Indexer: Michele Clark
Design: Design Resources Unit
Production Controller: Neil Dickson
Sales Promotion Executive: Kathy Crawford

Laparoscopic hysterectomy and oophorectomy:

A practical manual and colour atlas

Jeffrey H Phipps
BSc, MD, MRCOG
Consultant Gynaecologist,
The George Eliot Hospital, Nuneaton,
Warwickshire, UK

Foreword by

B Victor Lewis
MD, FRCS, FRCOG
President, British Society
of Gynaecological Endoscopy

Illustrations by

Peter Cox
RDD, MMAA, AIMI

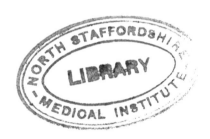

Churchill Livingstone
EDINBURGH LONDON MADRID MELBOURNE
NEW YORK AND TOKYO 1993

CHURCHILL LIVINGSTONE
Medical Division of Longman Group UK Limited

Distributed in the United States of America by
Churchill Livingstone Inc., 650 Avenue of the
Americas, New York, N.Y. 10011, and by associated
companies, branches and representatives throughout
the world.
© Longman Group UK Limited 1993

First published 1993
  Reprinted 1993

ISBN 0-443-04929-7

British Library of Cataloguing in Publication Data
A catalogue record for this book is available from
the British Library.

Library of Congress Cataloging in Publication Data
A catalog record for this book is available from the
Library of Congress.

The
publisher's
policy is to use
**paper manufactured
from sustainable forests**

Printed in Singapore

CONTENTS

CONTRIBUTORS

Medhat Hassanaien MB BS
Registrar, Obstetrics and Gynaecology,
The George Eliot Hospital, Nuneaton,
Warwickshire, UK

Michael John MB BS, MRCOG
Registrar, Obstetrics and Gynaecology,
The George Eliot Hospital, Nuneaton,
Warwickshire, UK

Peter J. Lefley MB BS, MRCGP
General Practitioner, Castle Mead Medical Centre,
Hill Street, Hinckley, Leicestershire, UK

Richard Miller MD, FFARCS
Consultant Anaesthetist and Director of
Intensive Care, The George Eliot Hospital,
Nuneaton, Warwickshire, UK

FOREWORD

Until recently, gynaecologists had only two methods of removing the uterus by either vaginal or abdominal hysterectomy, often combined with bilateral salpingo-oophorectomy. The gynaecological surgeon now has more options because there are three additional operations, namely laparoscopic assisted vaginal hysterectomy (LAVH), laparoscopic hysterectomy and the supra-cervical laparoscopic hysterectomy as described by Semm. New operative techniques need full evaluation, and the fact that they are technically possible is no indication for their performance. There is no substitute for care in selecting patients, and meticulous post-operative follow-up, with detailed records of complications. This well-illustrated practical manual emphasises the importance of patient selection, and lists the patients who are unsuitable for laparoscopic hysterectomy. There is particular emphasis on the technical aspects of the operation because high-technology equipment is required and, unless care is taken, problems can arise with the TV camera, with impaired clarity of the television image, and there can be difficulties in stopping bleeding, with either bipolar diathermy or staples. A number of original but practical technical advances are described, particularly elevation of the abdominal wall, by the 'C' retractor, so that vision can be maintained, even though the pneumo-peritoneum disappears when the vaginal vault is opened, and the use of illuminated ureteric catheters.

The main technical complication besides haemorrhage is damage to the bladder and ureter. Illuminated stents inserted into the ureters through a cystoscope means that the course of the pelvic ureter can be identified at all times, which is of especial value in the presence of endometriosis or chronic pelvic sepsis. This means that risk of damage to a ureter when the uterine arteries are clamped is substantially reduced. Drainage of the pelvis has not hitherto been emphasised in laparoscopic surgery, and I am delighted that Jeffrey Phipps has emphasised the importance of drains, especially if there is oozing from the pelvic side wall.

I welcome this well-written and highly-illustrated manual. It should be essential reading for all surgeons attempting to perform laparoscopically assisted vaginal hysterectomy, and should help them complete the operation with minimal complications and without excessive operating theatre time.

B V Lewis MD, FRCS, FRCOG
PRESIDENT BRITISH SOCIETY OF GYNAECOLOGICAL ENDOSCOPY

x

PREFACE

Endoscopic, particularly laparoscopic, surgery has now advanced to a degree where it is technically feasible to perform almost any operation previously requiring laparotomy. There has been what amounts to a revolution in the field of gynaecological surgery, partly due to the conception of new approaches to old surgical procedures, and partly due to the availability of highly sophisticated instrumentation and imaging systems. This is certainly true for laparoscopic hysterectomy and oophorectomy. What started as a novel surgical curio is rapidly becoming widely available to patients. In view of this, it is vital that this new surgical practice is carefully monitored and certainly audited. Much (healthy) scepticism exists concerning laparoscopic hysterectomy in particular, and the question 'how is it any better than vaginal hysterectomy?' is probably the one most often asked. The point is that the laparoscopic approach should not, and is not, intended to be a substitute for vaginal surgery; it is a substitute for open abdominal surgery in certain cases. For example, where oophorectomy is co-indicated. Those skilled in vaginal surgery often protest that it is possible to remove the ovaries vaginally, if necessary. This may well be true on occasion. In the real world, however, most would agree that '... and bilateral salpingoophorectomy' is usually appended to 'total abdominal hysterectomy'.

The second major concern about these new procedures is the length of the operation. One often hears of a laparoscopic total hysterectomy and bilateral salpingo-oophorectomy requiring two, three or more hours to complete. This need not necessarily be the case. With practice, the operation can usually be completed in around 70 minutes (or less in uncomplicated cases), provided the precepts of Doyen are adhered to: the minimum number of instruments consistent with safe and efficient surgery should be employed. There is never any need to, for example, coagulate with one modality (e.g. Nd YAG laser), and cut with another (e.g. carbon dioxide laser). Straightforward application of endoscopic staples and combined cutting/coagulating diathermy-armed scissors are all that is required. Alternatives to staples are cheaper, but prolong the operation and in some cases are less safe. Also of relevance to operation time is the question of the ureters. There is little doubt that one of the most common complications of laparoscopic hysterectomy is ureteric injury. Meticulous identification of the ureters by dissection and isolation is very time-consuming indeed. In those cases where ureteric anatomy is a cause for concern, the placing of transilluminating ureteric stents for identification is safe, effective and requires less than two minutes (with practice).

Finally, it is hoped that the experience and practice that stand behind the techniques detailed in this volume will help the reader to develop a safe and efficient technique, and to avoid as many pitfalls as possible.

J.H.P.   Nuneaton, 1992

ACKNOWLEDGEMENTS

My sincere thanks to the following:

B Victor Lewis MD, FRCS, FRCOG
President of the British Society for Gynaecological
Endoscopy and Consultant Gynaecological Surgeon,
whose vision, foresight and enthusiasm have been
largely responsible for the introduction of many
aspects of minimally invasive surgery into British
gynaecological practice.

John Scullion
Medical Photographer, Nuneaton Hospitals, for superb
photographic support.

Victor Kenyon FRCOG
Consultant Obstetrician and Gynaecologist, friend and
colleague, for his unending support and especially for
relieving me of many of the general burdens of work,
which has enabled me to pursue the clinical practice
and research so vital to the production of this book.

**The Management of George Eliot Hospital and
North East Warwickshire District Health Authority**
Chairman Geoffrey Jackson JP, CBE, Peter Stansbie,
John Townsend, David Thomas, Diane Kent, Sue Farr
and Peter Rock et al, without whose support and
imagination the clinical, teaching and research facility
for gynaecological minimally invasive surgery now
assembled at The George Eliot Hospital would never
have materialised.

J.H.P.   Nuneaton, 1992

INTRODUCTION

While controversy rages over whether or not laparoscopic hysterectomy or, to use the more widely used term, laparoscopically assisted vaginal hysterectomy (LAVH) is a valid operation, it seemed appropriate to produce a concise, practical manual of how to actually perform these techniques, for those who are convinced of their value. This book is for those who wish to *do*, rather than debate, this type of surgery.

With the increasing interest in oophorectomy both for prophylaxis against ovarian malignancy and as an adjunct to the treatment of breast cancer, the laparoscopic approach is becoming widely accepted as being that of choice, and so has been included in this book.

The laparoscopic approach to hysterectomy and oophorectomy has gained popularity in some centres in the US and Europe (Nezhat et al 1992, Bruhat et al 1991, Minelli et al 1991) and has been used for a wide range of conditions including stage I ovarian cancer (Reich 1989). Minelli (1991) advocates the laparoscopic route in preference to the unassisted vaginal route in cases where 'entero-uterine adhesions are present, adnexectomy is indicated, when the uterus is large, mobility poor or there is associated narrowing of the vaginal canal'. Contraindications to laparoscopic hysterectomy are few, but most authorities would include: uterine size greater than 12 weeks' gestation; intrauterine and ovarian malignancy beyond stage I; and where density of pelvic adhesions makes safe dissection of bowel and urinary tract impossible. It is possible, however, to pretreat with luteinising hormone releasing-hormone analogues to reduce fibroid size prior to surgery. It is also possible to morcellate the uterus laparoscopically after hysterectomy and extract it either transabdominally or vaginally, but this is time-consuming and makes histological examination difficult or impossible.

An increasing number of teaching courses in the UK are encouraging 'hands-on' practice and dissemination of these advanced laparoscopic procedures. The availability of disposable endoscopic stapling devices such as the Multifire Endo GIA™ 30 stapler (Auto Suture Company, Ascot, UK) has made dividing tissues and achieving haemostasis simultaneous, quick and relatively easy. The need to master difficult and lengthy laparoscopic suturing techniques is thereby reduced or obviated. The disadvantage of using such instruments is cost – a disposable stapler with four cartridges (required to divide and seal the infundibulopelvic ligaments and the uterine artery pedicles during total hysterectomy and bilateral salpingo-oophorectomy) costs approximately £390.00 ($700) at the time of writing.

While those skilled in vaginal surgery would argue that the laparoscopic approach has no advantage over simple vaginal hysterectomy, the same argument cannot be applied to hysterectomy with bilateral salpingo-oophorectomy. Although it may sometimes prove possible to excise the ovaries vaginally where sufficient descent exists, it is often impossible because the ovaries lie high in the pelvis. Laparoscopic oophorectomy alone has been extensively reported (Johns 1991, Nezhat et al 1991), but little has appeared in the literature concerning combined laparoscopic hysterectomy and bilateral oophorectomy.

This manual is *not* a presentation of various opinions and techniques of advanced laparoscopic surgery. It is, rather, a 'no-nonsense' guide to the practicalities of performing laparoscopic removal of the uterus and ovaries using straightforward techniques and equipment, with the minimum of 'frills'. Few 'alternative methods' of performing a particular stage of a particular operation will be found; what is presented is didactic and is based on the experience of the author. For example, the techniques described use staples, monopolar diathermy scissors and bipolar coagulation almost exclusively. That is not to say that the same operations cannot be performed using, for example, endoscopic sutures and lasers. However, it does mean that after due examination of alternative technologies, the ones detailed in this book have been selected because we believe they are the safest, most straightforward and most efficient, from both a surgical and a biomechanical perspective.

We have chosen to use the term 'laparoscopic hysterectomy' rather than 'laparoscopically assisted vaginal hysterectomy' (LAVH) for two reasons. The first is that LAVH suggests that the procedure is in reality a vaginal hysterectomy made a little easier by simple laparoscopic division of the superior pedicles. Although it is perfectly possible to use the technique to perform such operations, it is both inappropriate and unnecessarily costly to approach hysterectomy laparoscopically when the simple vaginal route would suffice. Laparoscopic surgery is expensive and, if resources are to be used efficiently, valid indications must exist before the laparoscopic route is chosen. If the technique is applied to suitable cases, it is by no means the case that a simple vaginal procedure would be appropriate. If oophorectomy is indicated, or if vaginal access is very poor, then vaginal hysterectomy may prove to be inappropriate, difficult or impossible.

The second reason for preferring the shorter term is literary. The indication for the laparoscopic approach may often be that oophorectomy is coindicated with hysterectomy. While advocates of vaginal surgery may sometimes be able to perform simultaneous oophorectomy vaginally, it is equally often the case that oophorectomy is impossible because the ovaries lie high in the pelvis. The term 'laparoscopically assisted vaginal hysterectomy and bilateral salpingo-oophorectomy' is unwieldy and so has been avoided.

It has been suggested that operations which include laparoscopic division of the uterine artery be termed 'laparoscopic hysterectomy', and those where the uterine artery is dealt with vaginally 'laparoscopically assisted vaginal hysterectomy'. It may be the case that this distinction will become accepted terminology but, for the present, 'laparoscopic hysterectomy', specifying method of uterine artery division, seems a clear and simple description.

Presented in this book is both evidence to support the contention that laparoscopic hysterectomy and oophorectomy either together or separately are useful and valid operations, and data on our experience of over 200 operations performed. The techniques are not without complications, notably ureteric injury and haemorrhage, and it is hoped that these may be avoided as much as possible by other surgeons taking advantage of the experience we have gained. The techniques described have evolved continuously and have been repeatedly revised in response to difficulties or complications as they have arisen. Each operation is described in considerable detail with accompanying endoscopic photographs and explanatory line drawings.

This manual is *not*, however, intended to be a substitute for proper training, but as an adjunct. The ideal way of learning any surgery is probably in the apprentice tradition, where the learner spends considerable time dogging the steps of the teacher and in time acquires the appropriate practical skills. For many surgeons this will, of course, be impossible, especially for those already in senior positions. Given that this is the case, intensive training courses are a practical, although less than ideal, alternative and there are now a considerable number of these on offer. If complication rates are to be kept to a minimum, it seems sensible that those embarking on advanced endoscopic surgery should be as fully trained as possible. It is hoped that this short manual will help.

A chapter is included on anaesthetic aspects of advanced laparoscopic surgery, and should be of particular interest to the growing number of anaesthetists who find themselves confronted with caring for patients undergoing lengthy endoscopic procedures. The implications of prolonged pneumo-peritoneum and Trendelenburg positioning are of particular note.

Finally, an 'extra' chapter is included which outlines the primary health care perspective on these relatively new procedures, written by a GP known inter-nationally for first introducing quality assurance systems (British Standard 5750, ISO 9000) into general practice. Surgeons would do well to read this section carefully; although it will not contribute to enhancing endoscopic surgical skills, it provides an invaluable insight into referral rationale and mechanism in general practice without whose patient referrals the gynaecologists skills go for naught.

If these advanced techniques are to become genuinely useful, widely practised operations to the benefit of the community, rather than surgical curios of the academically privileged, a wider view is needed. Virtually *any* operation is possible through the laparoscope, but what of the wider implications in terms of resource management and impact on the community at large? Surely these questions are as important as which are the optimal types of surgical instruments or diathermy generators? It is hoped that this broad approach will enable not only surgeons but colleagues in primary health care to appraise laparoscopic hysterectomy and oophorectomy with insight.

PATIENT SELECTION AND INDICATIONS FOR SURGERY

Selecting patients for laparoscopic hysterectomy and/or oophorectomy is no different from any other surgery – there must be suitable indication(s), without overwhelming contraindications. A balance must be achieved when selecting patients for these procedures, and it is wise never to *guarantee* a laparoscopic operation, but to emphasise that the possibility of laparotomy exists in cases of technical difficulty or intraoperative complication. On the one hand, attempting difficult surgery (obesity, severe adhesive disease or endometriosis) during the early part of the learning curve is not good practice. On the other hand, it is quite wrong merely to staple the upper pedicle in a patient where a simple vaginal hysterectomy would suffice in an effort to pay lip service to making the procedure 'laparoscopic'. This is a waste of resources and only fuels the lobby to brand laparoscopic hysterectomy as an 'expensive gimmick'. Indeed, this very epithet is the planned title (as an interrogative) of a forthcoming national meeting planned for the Royal College of Obstetricians and Gynaecologists (R. Garry, personal communication).

Once the decision has been made that
a. hysterectomy and/or oophorectomy is necessary
b. the patient wishes to avoid laparotomy
c. simple vaginal hysterectomy is considered inappropriate because oophorectomy is coindicated, pelvic adhesive disease exists or the uterus is enlarged to a degree where the upper pedicles would be likely to prove problematic were the simple vaginal route attempted
d. the appropriate skills and resources exist for attempting the laparoscopic route

then this approach is appropriate in the following circumstances.

1. WHEN OOPHORECTOMY ALONE IS INDICATED

Laparoscopic oophorectomy alone is indicated either when disease exists in the ovaries or as an adjunct in the treatment of premenopausal breast cancer. In the latter case, where the ovaries are healthy, the operation is relatively simple. They are excised, then either removed in a tissue retrieval bag via the abdomen or the pouch of Douglas transvaginally, or morcellated/liquidised and removed transabdominally. Excision of ovarian cysts may be achieved laparoscopically (where no suspicion of malignancy exists), but this may occasionally necessitate excision of the whole ovary.

Some authors advocate the treatment of stage I ovarian cancer laparoscopically (Reich 1989), but this is controversial and most endoscopic surgeons would limit their treatment to benign disease. Large simple ovarian cysts may be drained first followed by laparoscopic oophorectomy.

Contraindications to laparoscopic oophorectomy are those generally applied to laparoscopic surgery.

Severely obese women present a particular challenge. Gaining entry to the peritoneal cavity itself may be a problem, especially if the thickness of the abdominal wall is equal to, or exceeds, the length of the trochar and cannula. The incidence of inadvertent injection of carbon dioxide into the tissues of the abdominal wall is therefore higher, which makes subsequent peritoneal access even more difficult. Special extra-long (non-disposable) trochar/cannulae are available for dealing with this problem but, even so, instrument manipulation in very obese patients may be difficult or occasionally impossible. If the depth of the abdominal wall through which the hand instruments have to pass is 50% or more of the length of the shaft of the instrument, it is very difficult indeed to achieve the 'sweeping' movements required to perform surgery. The peritoneum and omentum invariably cause difficulty with access and operative visualisation because they tend to be replete with fat. The patient also presents problems to the anaesthetist, who finds that ventilation is difficult to maintain, especially with significant Trendelenburg tilt and splinting of the diaphragm due to prolonged pneumoperitoneum. General postoperative complications are also more common, particularly thromboembolic disease and infection. It is the practice of the author not to attempt advanced laparoscopic surgery on a patient who is more than 40% over her ideal bodyweight, but this may be somewhat over-generous.

2. WHEN LAPAROSCOPIC HYSTERECTOMY IS INDICATED BECAUSE BILATERAL OOPHORECTOMY IS COINDICATED

The laparoscopic route is preferred to the unassisted vaginal route when hysterectomy is indicated but there exists a coindication for oophorectomy. This may be because of the patient's age (usually taken as over 45 years, as prophylaxis against malignancy), severe refractory premenstrual syndrome (PMS), known or suspected non-malignant ovarian abnormality (e.g. cysts), severe cyclic pelvic pain or patient preference.

Contraindications are those stated for laparoscopic surgery in general, with the addition of uterine size: our practice is to limit the offer of laparoscopic surgery to 12 weeks' gestation size. While it is technically feasible to operate on almost *any* size of uterus, the complication rate (bleeding, injury to other intra-abdominal organs because of poor view) and operative time (reports of up to 6 hours are not uncommon) are usually considered unacceptable. If the isolated uterus has to be morcellated to any greater extent than simple bisection (vaginally) in order to negotiate the pelvic outlet, operative time is likely to be very long indeed, with all the attendant anaesthetic problems and post-operative risks.

3. WHEN LAPAROSCOPIC HYSTERECTOMY IS INDICATED BECAUSE VAGINAL ACCESS IS POOR

The same general indications for surgery exist: intractable dysfunctional bleeding (in our own practice usually those who are not satisfied with the outcome of medical therapy or endometrial ablation), symptomatic fibroadenomata (12 weeks' gestation size or smaller) and stage I endometrial carcinoma. Whilst some of those especially skilled in vaginal surgery would argue that vaginal access is *never* so poor that vaginal hysterectomy is impossible, many would agree that it may be a most difficult operation when the combination of narrow pubic arch, limited vaginal space and poor descent exists. Under these conditions, there is little doubt that laparoscopic hysterectomy is a somewhat easier option, and may therefore be safer if open abdominal hysterectomy is to be avoided.

Under these circumstances, the laparoscopic dissection may advance as far as desired, including the uterosacral ligaments and vaginal skin, such that no vaginal dissection is required at all. While this approach is used in Europe (J. Pouly, personal communication), in the opinion of the author it is never necessary to go beyond the uterine arteries and bladder laparoscopically. Proceeding beyond to the uterosacral ligaments and vaginal skin is time-consuming, potentially hazardous (because of the proximity of the ureters) and expensive in terms of both theatre time and disposable staples or endoscopic sutures. The vaginal skin and uterosacral ligaments are almost invariably accessible vaginally and, in those rare cases where they are not (for example in severe vaginal stenosis), it may be preferable to adopt the open abdominal route, although *total* laparoscopic hysterectomy is practised in a number of centres with success.

3

INSTRUMENTATION AND EQUIPMENT

Hand instruments

Staples, sutures and diathermy

Imaging equipment and insufflation

Elementary fault diagnosis and rectification

There is currently available a bewildering variety of hand instruments, video equipment, lasers of astonishing variety, intra-abdominal aqua-dissectors and ultrasonic tissue liquidisers, electrosurgical units with and without argon 'beamer' facility – the list is almost endless. Those embarking on the techniques described here may receive the impression that very large sums of money are needed to equip an operating theatre for laparoscopic surgery, if they attend any of the major meetings concerned with minimally invasive surgery.

Although there is no doubt that a good quality imaging system and set of instruments is required, by and large many of the devices on offer are very much 'icing on the cake' and are not essential for these techniques. For example, in the opinion of the author, lasers of any variety do not offer significant advantages over diathermy either for dissection or coagulation. While it may well be the case that the neodymium–yttrium–aluminium–garnet (Nd YAG) or excimer laser is the instrument of choice for ablating endometriosis, or the carbon dioxide laser that of choice for adhesiolysis, these expensive devices are not essential for performing laparoscopic hysterectomy or oophorectomy. A simple diathermy machine capable of delivering both monopolar cutting and coagulation current and bipolar coagulation current is perfectly adequate for all dissection and haemostasis.

The range of hand instruments available is very extensive indeed, but again, very few are essential in practice. It should be emphasised that the list of essential instruments detailed here is a personal one.

HAND INSTRUMENTS

Hand instruments must be of high quality. Although this sounds obvious, it is surprising how many articles of inferior quality are available.

All instruments should be insulated and capable of carrying diathermy via a standard-gauge connector. There are, at the time of writing, several different types of connector used. It is essential that a single diathermy supply lead for monopolar current and another for bipolar coagulation are employed rather than having to change constantly from one type of lead to another intraoperatively.

A diathermy lead unconnected to any instrument which has inadvertently been left connected to the electrosurgical generator may cause severe burns if the socket lies on the patient. Diathermy active instruments must *always* be kept sheathed in an insulated container when not in use. The appropriate power settings for any individual generator will be decided upon with experience.

In the opinion of the author, the following instruments are essential:

1. Heavy graspers, self-locking (1)
2. Heavy graspers, non-self-locking (1)
3. Snipe-nosed graspers, non-self-locking (1)
4. Scissors, hook-nosed (1)
5. Scissors, straight or curved (1)
6. Needle point diathermy (1)
7. Laparoscopic needle holder (1) (Fig. 3.1)
8. Wash/suck device – an excellent version is available with the addition of diathermy (1) (Fig. 3.2)
9. Trochar and cannulae, 5 mm, 10 mm and 12 mm – unless disposable units are to be used, which, although preferable, are expensive (2 of each)
10. Standard set of instruments for completing the vaginal dissection

Items 1–5 should ideally have rotatable operating heads such that tissue may be clamped or divided in any plane whilst maintaining a comfortable hand position.

The major advantage of using disposable trochar and cannulae is that they are available in a 12 mm size to suit the laparoscopic stapling device (see above), and reducing seals are available such that 5 mm hand instruments may be used with the same cannula. This avoids the need to change the cannula constantly according to the diameter of the instrument in use. Furthermore, the disposable cannulae may be used with a securing device which prevents the cannula slipping too far in or out of the abdomen (Figs 3.3 and 3.4).

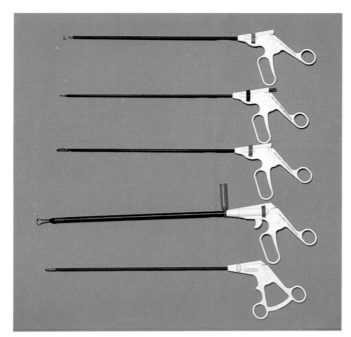

Fig. 3.1 **Laparoscopic hand instruments.**
Those shown are disposable with rotatable operating ends
(Auto Suture Company).

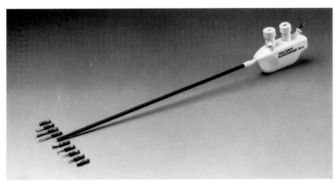

Fig. 3.2 **Wash/suction device (5 mm), diathermy-armed.**
Surgiwand™ irrigation/suction device (Auto Suture Company).

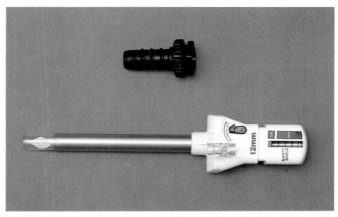

Fig. 3.3 **Disposable 12 mm trochar/cannula with abdominal wall
fixing device** (Surgiport™ and Surgigrip™, Auto Suture Company).

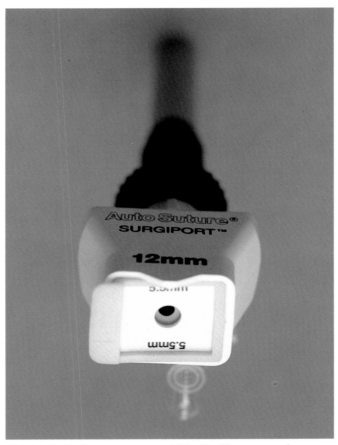

Fig. 3.4 **Reducing converter seal fitted to 12 mm cannula.**

If the uterine artery pedicle is to be taken vaginally (in those cases where vaginal access is good – see above), the haemostatic clamps for ligating and dividing the uterine artery pedicle should be longitudinally ridged, straight and non-toothed, such as Rogers or Zeppelin clamps (Fig. 3.5). The reason for this is that it is necessary to make certain that the uterine artery pedicle is clamped up to and including the inferior margin of the laparoscopic dissection line, otherwise bleeding may occur from the free tissue between the vaginal and the laparoscopic dissection (see section on complications, below). Application of the haemostatic clamp to the uterine artery may be difficult, particularly if descent is poor, and it is vital that excessive traction is not employed. The upper small branches of the uterine artery are easily torn and may be very difficult indeed to arrest, particularly if the vessels have sheared off flush with the pelvic side wall. An instrument is therefore needed which will slide easily over the tissues without snagging (hence non-toothed), and is guaranteed not to slip (hence longitudinally ridged).

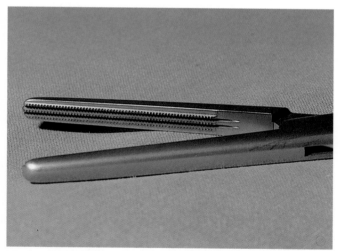

Fig. 3.5 **Clamping faces of Rogers haemostatic clamps used for vaginal dissection.**

STAPLES, SUTURES AND DIATHERMY

Tissue dissection may be achieved laparoscopically either by mechanical means (scissors), electrically (diathermy) or by laser. As already stated, it is the belief of the author that, as far as the applications discussed in this book are concerned, lasers have no significant advantages over diathermy, and they are exceedingly expensive. A special set of instruments is also required to deliver the laser energy into the abdomen. In practice, there is little difference between the cutting power of the carbon dioxide laser and that of needle point cutting diathermy, just as there is little difference between the coagulation and penetration power of the Nd YAG laser and that of coagulation diathermy. Although other workers have widely stated that various lasers are the instruments of choice, they will not be discussed further in the present volume.

Similarly, although aqua-dissection is a useful technique in several areas of laparoscopic surgery, it is not essential to the present application. The aqua-dissector (Wisap, Germany) is a high-pressure, low-volume pump device which delivers a jet of water or saline via a fine-bore laparoscopic needle. The force of the fluid jet is capable of separating tissues, but usually only where the plane of dissection is loose and unscarred. The bladder, for example, may be freed from the anterior aspect of the uterus after the peritoneal flap is raised by directing the jet at the loose areolar tissue which is encountered. This dissection may easily be achieved by simple scissors and blunt dissection alone, however, and aqua-dissection will therefore not be discussed further.

Haemostasis likewise may be achieved in a number of different ways. Diathermy is the cheapest and, for some applications, the most suitable. The safest method of delivering coagulation diathermy is by using the bipolar mode, such that current flows only through the structure grasped rather than through surrounding tissues (Fig. 3.6). If monopolar diathermy is used, especially at high power, then heating of non-target tissues may occur as current flows through adjacent structures (Fig. 3.7). There is also the risk of arcing from the instrument to adjacent structures (notably bowel), as the high voltage seeks a path to earth as a result of the increased impedance of the target tissue as desiccation occurs (Fig. 3.8).

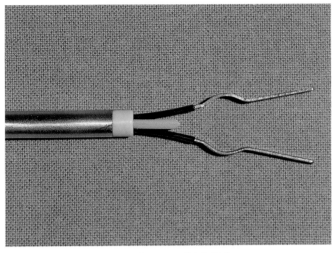

Fig. 3.6 **Bipolar diathermy forceps** (Wolf, UK).

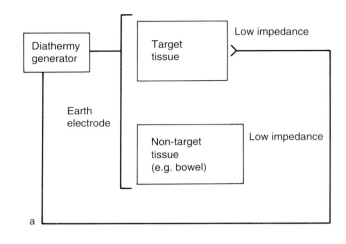

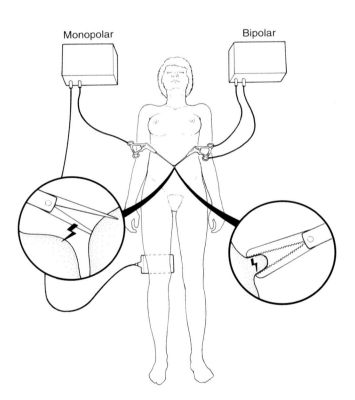

Fig. 3.7 **Bipolar and monopolar diathermy current flow.**

Fig. 3.8 **Increased risk of arcing to non-target tissue with increasing target tissue impedance after desiccation.**

The disadvantages of using diathermy alone for haemostasis are, firstly, that very high temperatures are developed in the heated tissues, often in excess of 120°C (personal research). Even if bipolar diathermy is used, this is a sufficiently high temperature to drive a temperature gradient such that adjacent tissues may be heated to histotoxic levels (above approximately 50°C for more than a few seconds, Hahn 1989). Experimentally, thermometry probes placed at regular intervals from a bipolar diathermy probe during electrocoagulation of parametrial tissue in open hysterectomy volunteers reveal an alarming temperature rise in adjacent tissues (data submitted for publication) (Fig. 3.9). This is particularly hazardous when using diathermy on the infundibulopelvic or uterosacral ligaments, because of the proximity of the ureter, with the consequent risk of thermal injury, necrosis and fistulation.

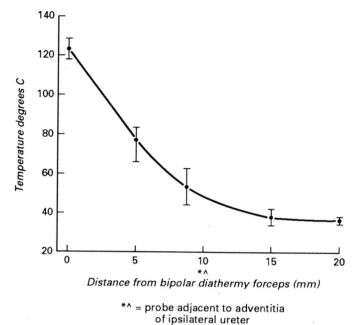

*^ = probe adjacent to adventitia
of ipsilateral ureter

n = 3 (vertical bars represent temperature range
for all patients)

Fig. 3.9 **Temperature gradient during use of bipolar diathermy forceps.** Temperatures plotted represent peak values recorded.

The second problem is that, in the case of large vessels, even if haemostasis may appear secure after heating, bleeding may occur later as a result of the heated tissue necrosing. If pressure within larger vessels is sufficient and thrombosis has not occurred, the seal may break down, resulting in haemorrhage.

Monopolar coagulation diathermy is, however, ideal for securing haemostasis in small vessels and is particularly suited to use with endoscopic scissors. An excellent method of dividing the bladder peritoneum, for example, is the use of diathermy-armed scissors. It is important that the delivery of diathermy is timed correctly. The scissor blades must be in good contact, with pressure applied such that the blades 'sink' into the tissue slightly before current is applied. The reason for this is that if the current is applied before contact with tissue then arcing is bound to occur between the narrowest part of the instrument (i.e. the cutting edges) and the target tissue (Fig. 3.10). This results in rapid blunting or even seizure of the instrument.

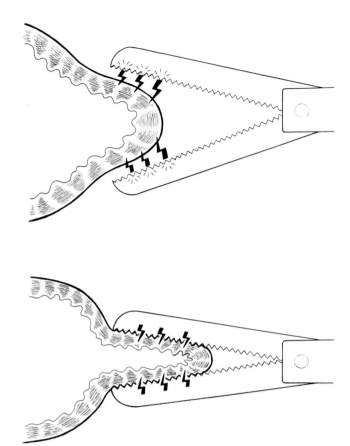

Fig. 3.10 **Diathermy arcing to scissor cutting edges with consequent blunting due to premature diathermy activation.**

One final method of thermally coagulating tissue is the use of a simple ohmically heated probe/forceps which operates at around 100°C, first described by Semm (Endo-Coagulator™, Wisap, Germany). This device is very useful for arresting bleeding from large 'raw' surface areas and medium-size vessels, and operates by simply heating tissues to a degree where protein denaturation occurs, including clotting of blood. Indeed, the great Professor Kurt Semm forbids the use of diathermy under any circumstances in his unit because of the risks attached to its use and the relative safety of the Endo-Coagulator™ (personal communication). The disadvantages of this technique are that larger vessels cannot be adequately controlled (without the same risks as with diathermy of tissue sloughing and later haemorrhage); it is time-consuming and relatively imprecise in its action compared to diathermy. 'Endo-coagulation' relies upon a simple thermal gradient for heating tissue, rather than developing heat within the target tissue itself, and is therefore slower and results in a rather poorly defined area of coagulation.

Laparoscopic suturing has the advantage of relatively low cost (compared to staples), but the disadvantage of being somewhat more difficult to master than diathermy or stapling techniques. There are basically three types of laparoscopic suture available.

In loop devices, a pre-tied loop in the form of a 'lasso' is introduced into the abdomen then tightened from outside, which may only be used to secure haemostasis in situations where the tissue is 'open-ended' (Fig. 3.11). Such a loop cannot be used to secure haemostasis very easily where tissues are continuous, i.e. with no free border to allow placement of the loop – the infundibulopelvic ligament, for example (Fig. 3.12).

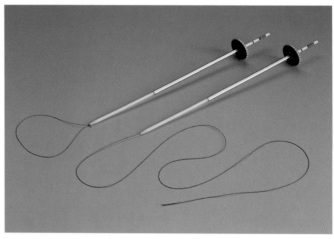

Fig. 3.11 **Endoscopic loop device (left) and disposable extra-corporeal knotting suture ligature (Surgiwip™) (right)** (Auto Suture Company).

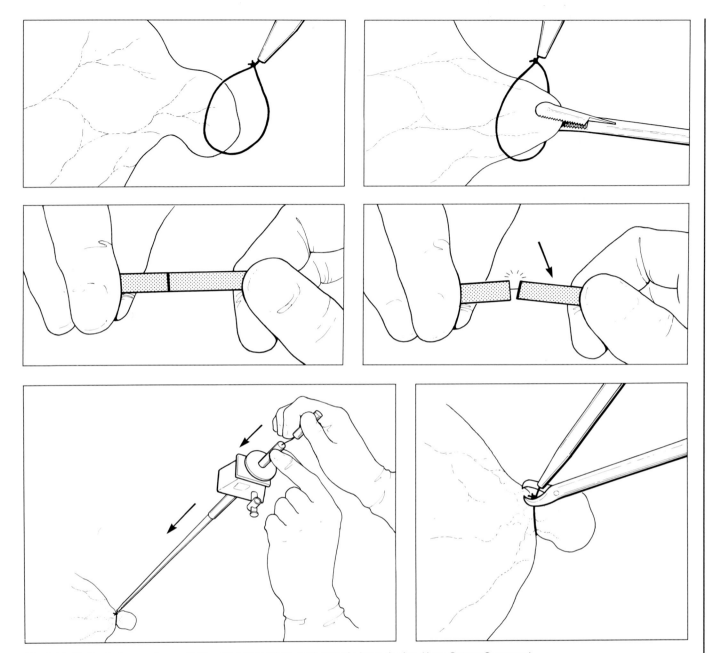

Fig. 3.12 **Method of securing pedicle using Surgitic™ endoscopic loop device** (Auto Suture Company).

The second type of suture is little different from a normal bonded suture, although 'ski-shaped' needles are easier to handle inside the abdomen than either straight or curved needles and are supplied with short thread. Purpose-designed laparoscopic needle holders are essential for using such sutures and the knot is tied inside the abdomen – a feat which requires considerable practice! These are ideal for securing haemostasis where bleeding originates from a flat surface – for example the pelvic side-wall, a situation where diathermy or laser may mean risk to the ureter and staples or loops are not applicable.

Finally, there are a number of ingenious devices available which allow sutures to be placed within the abdomen in the same way as previously described, but the knot is tied *outside* the abdomen and then pushed down a trochar with a special knot-pusher to be tightened at the distal end at the target site (extracorporeal knot tying, Figs 3.11 and 3.13). This is a highly effective technique and is relatively cheap and straightforward. The disadvantage is that tissue 'bunching' occurs, sometimes making division of large pedicles difficult, as the suture sinks into the tissues and becomes difficult to identify prior to tissue division. Inadvertent division of the suture which has just been placed is not an unusual occurrence.

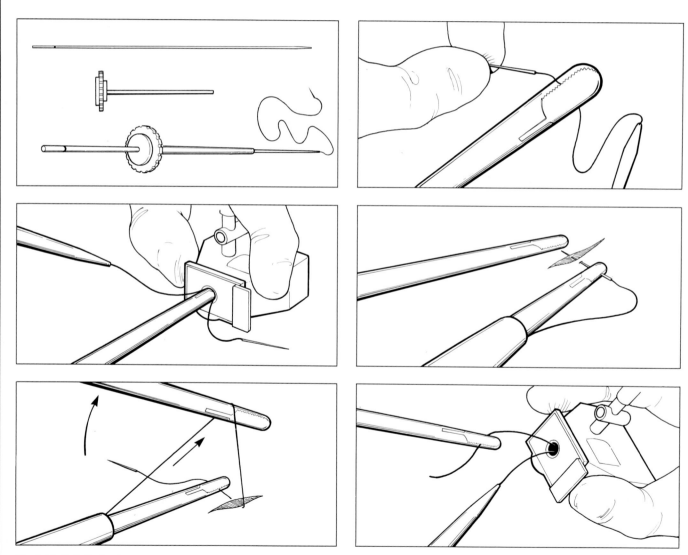

Fig. 3.13 **Detail of extracorporeal knot tying using Surgiwip**™ **suturing device** (Auto Suture Company).

There can be little doubt that, with the wide availability of laparoscopic stapling techniques, advanced laparoscopic surgery has become safer, faster and open to a wider group of surgeons.

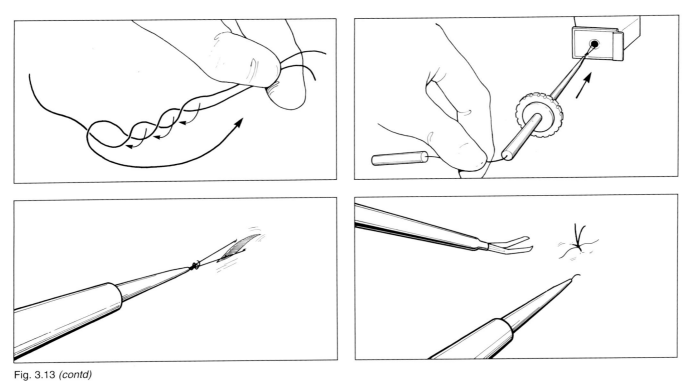

Fig. 3.13 *(contd)*

Probably the most useful of the stapling devices to the gynaecological surgeon at the time of writing is the Multifire Endo GIA™ stapler (Auto Suture Company; Fig. 3.14). This is a 12 mm diameter device which is capable of clamping and dividing tissue over a length of up to 30 mm, simultaneously securing haemostasis. When fired, the stapler delivers two triple staggered rows of titanium staples into the tissues, then drives a knife blade between the rows to divide them (Fig. 3.15). If correctly applied (see section on basic fault diagnosis and rectification, below) the result is invariably dry, clean edges which are haemostatically secure. One advantage of this device is that it is possible to place and clamp the jaws over the tissues atraumatically, allowing for repositioning without tissue damage if necessary. This is vital when operating in the vicinity of the ureter (see section on ureteric injury in Chapter 7).

The staple cartridge is available in two 'closure sizes': 2.5 mm (white colour-coded) and 3.5 mm (blue colour-coded) (Fig. 3.15). The staples in both cartridges are identical; it is only the closure height that varies, i.e. how much tissue they penetrate before they meet the anvil of the staple gun and are formed into a 'B' shape. This allows tissues of different thicknesses to be dealt with (Fig 3.16). If staples of inappropriately large height are used, haemostasis will fail due to poor tissue compression. If staples of inappropriately small closure height are used, they will meet the anvil before full-thickness tissue penetration has occurred and haemostasis will fail because the staples have closed before penetrating the full thickness of the target tissue. The use of the Endo Gauge™ (Auto Suture Company) allows tissue thickness to be measured prior to stapling (Fig. 3.17) although, in the opinion of the author, for the experienced surgeon this is rarely necessary. The reason for this is that the tissues encountered in laparoscopic hysterectomy/oophorectomy are invariably of a thickness that requires the 3.5 mm (blue cartridge) staple. However, it is suggested that the surgeon should *always* measure tissue thickness prior to staple application until experience dictates otherwise.

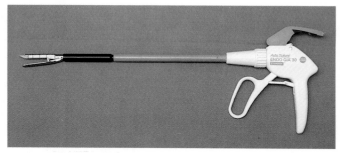

Fig. 3.14 **Multifire Endo GIA**™ **30 stapler** (Auto Suture Company).

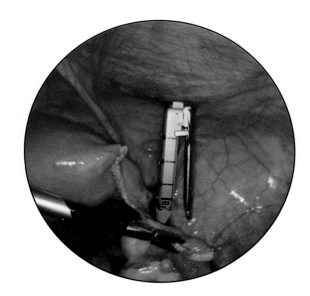

Fig. 3.15 **Detail of operating end of Multifire Endo GIA**™ **stapler.**

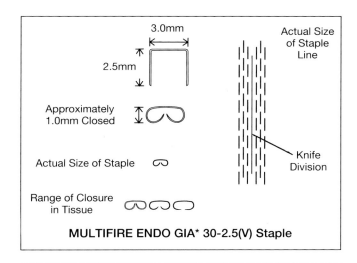

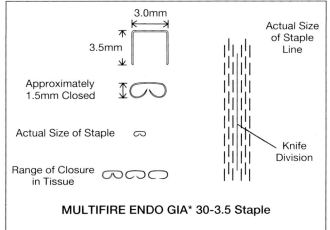

Fig. 3.16 **Detail of staple size and closure height of (above) the Multifire Endo GIA™ 30V (2.5) staple and (below) the Multifire Endo GIA™ 30 (3.5) staple.**

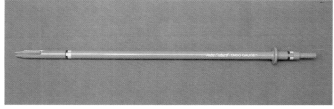

Fig. 3.17 **Tissue thickness gauge** (Endo Gauge™, Auto Suture Company).

While it is possible to use stapling devices for the vaginal dissection, this adds expense to an already expensive procedure; traditional suturing techniques are adequate.

There is now a 60 mm device available from the same company as the Multifire Endo GIA™ 30 stapler (Fig. 3.18), but its role in gynaecological surgery is not yet clear. Certainly, a device which is capable of dividing and effecting haemostasis simultaneously over double the length of the Multifire Endo GIA™ 30 stapler is appealing, but one suspects that the risk of ureteric injury, unless adequate precautions are taken, might be increased.

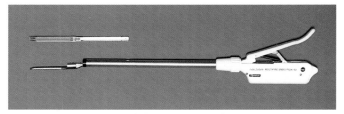

Fig. 3.18 **Multifire Endo GIA™ 60 mm stapler.**

One additional, although at the time of writing unproven, advantage of stapling is that the volume of ischaemic, and therefore necrosing, tissue remaining after control of the pedicle is minimal. The 'B' shape of the staple allows microvascular circulation to continue at the edge of the dissection line, such that even the very small volume of tissue distal to the staple line remains viable. The opposite is true when either diathermy or suturing techniques are used – significant volumes of non-viable tissue remain which must be reabsorbed, and certainly must provoke an inflammatory reaction. It may therefore be the case that operative recovery is improved by the use of staples, but at the present time this is conjecture.

IMAGING EQUIPMENT AND INSUFFLATION

There are now a number of companies producing excellent quality colour video monitoring equipment, some of which is better than others. The essential requirements of a suitable system are:

a. *Quality.* The quality of the image is all-important, and it is just as important that image quality is sustainable. When selecting equipment on demonstration, ensure that the image does not deteriorate after several hours' use. With some systems, as components begin to heat the image deteriorates.

b. *Reliability.* The system must be capable of tolerating the heavy usage and less than ideal treatment it is likely to encounter in theatre. The only way of ensuring this is to purchase only well-known equipment from reputable companies, where the service back-up is of high quality. It is essential that the company is able to offer an emergency 'repair or replace' service within 24–48 hours if problems are to be avoided in the event of component failure.

c. *Ease of use.* The equipment should be simple to use and should not require a specialist technician to operate it. Most importantly, the camera (or integrated telescope and camera in some systems) must be compact and lightweight. The camera/laparoscope operator is less likely to fatigue and fail in his duties if the instrument is easy to handle.

The essential components of a video system are:

a.   *The colour camera*
b.   *The camera control unit*
c.   *The light source.* This should be an automatically variable intensity unit, such that information from the camera is fed into the light source which then regulates its output to suit the current image conditions. The closer the laparoscope becomes to the tissues, the more light is reflected, and the output of the light source should reduce to avoid glare or 'white-out' of the image.
d.   *The colour monitor.* This should be of high pixel rating to give a grain-free image.
e.   *The video recorder.* For several reasons, it is essential that recording facilities are available, both to learn and to teach. There is little question that the format of choice is U-Matic, because the picture quality is unrivalled. The disadvantage is that the tape cannot be played on an ordinary VHS machine, but it is easily copied on to the more common format. Recording on VHS as the primary recording mode is generally unsatisfactory because of inferior picture quality compared to U-Matic.
f.   *The insufflator.* This should be a high-flow device. Laparoscopic surgery is impossible with the older low-flow (1 l.min^{-1}) machines used for diagnostic laparoscopy. A suitable machine should be capable of delivering at least 4 l.min^{-1} and preferably 9 l.min^{-1} in continuous-flow mode. Gas should be supplied directly from the cylinder, not from an internal reservoir tank which requires constant filling (Fig. 3.19).
g.   *Accessories.* It is important that the light-guide cable is of high quality, preferably fluid-filled and in good condition. Diathermy leads *must* be in good repair to avoid peripheral burns to the patient.

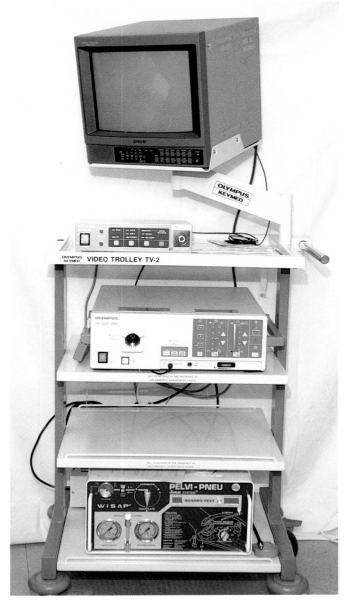

Fig. 3.19 **Typical imaging system. Note articulated monitor mounting which allows optimal placement for the surgical team.**

ELEMENTARY FAULT DIAGNOSIS AND RECTIFICATION

The majority of difficulties attributable to equipment failure are usually rectifiable by the operator, unless there is a genuine fault with a piece of equipment. In practice, the latter is rarely the case and problems with equipment are more often than not due to incorrect use or loose connections. The following is a brief guide to those common errors which may arise with endoscopic surgical equipment, and how they may be dealt with.

IMAGING AND VIDEO EQUIPMENT

1. Failure of any image to appear
Check that:
- all connections are tight and in the appropriate sockets
- appropriate 'routing' of the video signal is selected. On most systems there is the capability to select different outputs and inputs to/from the monitor
- the camera multipin plug is dry and clean and has not been submerged in sterilising fluid. This is *essential*, as severe damage to the camera may result if the plug becomes contaminated with water
- all units display a 'power on' light
- if several video formats are provided for on some of the component units (e.g. PAL, NTSC, SECAM), the correct mode is selected.

2. Blurred, out of focus or dark image
Check that:
- the end of the laparoscope is clean and dry. Misting of the laparoscope is by far the most common cause of a poor image. The instrument should be warm, and preferably used with an anti-misting agent such as Ultrastop. The carbon dioxide inflow should always be connected to one of the lower ports rather than the laparoscope port, since the inflowing gas is cold and promotes misting
- the camera is focused
- the auto-regulation connection lead is correctly in place between the camera control unit and the light source. Failure to make this connection may result in underexposure and a dark image
- The light-guide cable is the correct one, is in good condition and undamaged. If in doubt (with the more common fibreoptic cables), shine the output of the bare-ended cable on to a dark surface. The individual fibres of the light cable will be visible as bright dots; the appearance of patches without dots signifies that some of the fibres are broken and the cable should be replaced. A dark image results from a damaged light-guide cable. Light-guide cables are often available in several diameters for different applications (e.g. hysteroscopy and laparoscopy), although with interchangeable connectors. Use of a cable of inappropriately small diameter results in a dark image, especially when the distance between the end of the laparoscope and the tissues is long
- the light source is set to the correct output. Most machines function optimally on the 'automatic' setting.

3. Excessive smoke inside the peritoneal cavity
Although some insufflators are fitted with a gas recirculating and filtering mechanism, these are generally expensive and inessential. It is best not to generate excessive smoke in the first place: avoid intense heating of tissue by prolonged diathermy (or use of the carbon dioxide laser, which produces copious volumes of smoke). Blood and tissue coagulates at around 60°C; this temperature is rapidly achieved with bipolar diathermy and there is no need to 'blacken' tissues to achieve haemostasis. If the cavity *does* fill with smoke to an extent where vision is impaired, it is best to release the pneumoperitoneum completely and refill the abdomen with uncontaminated gas.

4. Failure of video recorder to record
Check that:
- all connectors are tight and in the correct sockets
- the machine is set to 'record', and from the appropriate source if multiple source selection is available on the machine
- the tape is not protected from accidental erasure.

If these simple measures fail, professional assistance will be required.

OTHER EQUIPMENT

Listed here are a number of common faults which have repeatedly shown up with equipment other than the imaging system, with simple remedies. The importance of having designated properly trained theatre staff cannot be overemphasised. In our centre, three of the nursing staff and two of the operating theatre technicians have taken a special interest and are fully familiar with the technology required for advanced endoscopic surgery, including instrument and imaging system care, routine servicing and elementary fault diagnosis.

1. Insufflation

Failure to establish or maintain insufflation may be due either to inadequate gas entering the abdomen (machine set incorrectly, gas cylinder empty, gas tubing kinked or gas tap partially or fully turned off at the cannula), or gas escaping from the abdomen at a rate exceeding that at which it can be replaced. Gas commonly leaks from around the cannulae (especially if overlarge incisions have been made), from the cannulae themselves (an unconnected gas tap inadvertently left switched on, or gas seals around the instruments in poor condition) or, if the vagina has been opened, transvaginally.

Overinsufflation is an uncommon problem, but is usually apparent to the anaesthetist in the first instance, because ventilation becomes difficult. This is invariably due to the insufflator being incorrectly set to an excessively high pressure.

2. Diathermy

As previously stated, diathermy settings suitable for a particular machine will be determined with experience. Minimal power consistent with efficient surgery should always be the aim in order to reduce the risk of burns to non-target tissues. Connections must be tight and dry, and the earth electrode properly sited. The patient must not come into contact with any earthed metallic surface, otherwise burns may result. It is *vital* that the distal end of any diathermy-armed laparoscopic instrument is fully and clearly visualised before being activated.

Bipolar diathermy generators are available with current flow meters built in. The purpose of this facility is to be able to judge when tissues are fully desiccated. When current flow is minimal (after prolonged diathermy), tissue impedance must therefore be maximal, i.e. with the minimum of water remaining in the tissue clamped. It is important that the generator is correctly connected and that the operator understands the principle of current monitoring.

Diathermy-armed instruments must always be sheathed when not in use, preferably with the diathermy generator on 'stand-by' mode. Inadvertent activation of diathermy-armed instruments inside the abdomen can lead to catastrophe.

3. Staplers

Provided the Multifire Endo GIA™ stapler is not overloaded with tissue, and a new disposable loading unit (DLU) is fitted correctly for each firing, this instrument operates reliably without problems. However, if incorrectly used, four common difficulties may occur: 1) failure of the jaws to open either before or after tissue stapling; 2) complete tissue transection does not occur (which may mean that a small bridge of tissue remains undivided between the two triple staple rows); 3) failure to fire at all; and 4) partial failure of haemostasis (almost always at the proximal margin of the staple line).

Failure of the jaws to open occurs most commonly because the hinge mechanism is not clear of the distal end of the cannula, so that the proximal end of the jaws is trapped in the cannula. Although this sounds obvious, and is easily cured by advancing the stapler until the proximal end is clear of the distal end of the cannula, it is a common cause of complaint. Alternatively, the jaws may – rarely – fail to open after tissue stapling, despite being clear of the end of cannula. This invariably happens because excessive tissue has been taken in one operation, fouling the hinge mechanism. The volume of tissue clamped should not be so great such that the proximal edge of the tissue to be divided impinges upon the hinge mechanism. There should be a gap of approximately 1 mm between the hinge mechanism and the leading edge of the tissue, which prevents fouling of the hinge and consequent jamming.

Should jamming occur, however, it is easily rectified. If the jaws will not open, despite the clamping lever being open and the jaws being clear of the end of cannula, the shaft of the instrument should be struck smartly with a metal instrument near to where the stapler enters the cannula. In our experience, the shock is always sufficient to release the jaws.

Failure of the stapler to fire, provided the trigger safety latch is disengaged, is invariably caused by the inadvertent loading of a used staple cartridge. The instrument will not allow the firing handle to close on a spent cartridge. This prevents transection of tissue without prior stapling and severe haemorrhage. Our practice is to discard used cartridges away from the instrument trolley so that mistakes cannot occur.

Failure to transect tissue completely (such that a tissue 'bridge' is left behind between the two staple lines) and failure of absolute haemostasis (almost invariably from the most proximal part of the dissection line) are caused by overloading the stapler with tissue. The 1 mm gap already described between the leading tissue edge and the hinge mechanism *must* be observed. If tissue is forced past the hinge bar (Fig. 3.20), no staples cover this area, and bleeding is the usual result. Prompt bipolar diathermy resolves the difficulty. Similarly, the knife mechanism is unable to cope with excessive tissue 'bunched' at the proximal end of the jaws of the instrument, and incomplete tissue transection is the result.

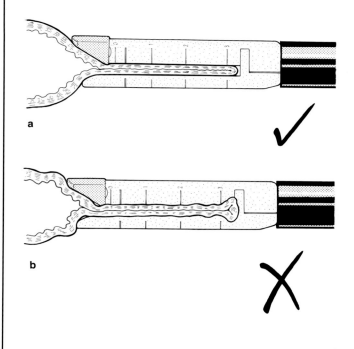

Fig. 3.20 Correct (a) and excessive (b) tissue loading of stapler. Excessive loading leads to loss of haemostasis and failure of tissue division.

Finally, care should be taken, when applying a second row of staples (for example, when securing the uterine artery after dissecting the infundibulopelvic ligament and urinary tract in hysterectomy) that staples do not excessively overlap. If staples are fired into tissue already bearing staples, they tend to become tangled and close imperfectly because they do not accurately strike the forming-anvil jaw of the instrument but are deflected from their proper course by the staples already there. This can lead to fouling of the stapler jaws with resultant jamming, or loss of haemostasis. It is usually of little consequence if two or three staples overlap, but care should be taken to site the second row of staples in such a way that the proximal end of the stapler jaws lies in the 'V' of the previous dissection and overlap is minimised.

It is worth noting that if staples are fired from part of the cartridge without intervening tissue, they are likely to remain trapped in the anvil of the instrument. This is not problematic, *provided* they are removed from the anvil prior to fitting the new cartridge. Failure to do so results in the staples of the next cartridge failing to close properly and possible loss of haemostasis.

4. Hand instruments

Very little can go wrong with these, except for slipping ratchets on self-locking forceps and similar devices, blunt scissors or blocked wash-suck devices and non-disposable trochar/cannulae. The first two can only be corrected by replacement, the other by regular and meticulous cleaning (unless disposable units are used). With growing experience, the surgeon will discover that expensive non-disposable scissors in particular become blunt and useless very quickly indeed, and are either difficult or impossible to re-sharpen. Repeated autoclave sterilisation of non-disposable hand instruments also eventually leads to compromise of the insulating plastic cover, which can lead to disaster if bowel, in particular, is inadvertently exposed to diathermy arcing because of imperfect insulation.

The experienced laparoscopic surgeon quickly discovers that with few exceptions, despite the best efforts of theatre staff, most non-disposable instruments eventually become worn and irretrievably contaminated by carbon, denatured blood, etc., with resulting impaired function. Disposable scissors, although expensive, are *always* sharp; tearing of tissue and consequent loss of haemostasis is therefore avoided.

4

ANAESTHESIA, PRE-OPERATIVE ASSESSMENT AND POSTOPERATIVE CARE

R. Miller

Minimally invasive surgery (MIS) is perhaps one of the most exciting developments in medicine in the last 50 years. As the new order of surgical expertise increases and instrument technology is refined, a virtual 'explosion' in video-controlled surgery may be anticipated. The trauma of open access for surgery – retraction, exposure and handling of viscera – is minimised, recovery is much faster and it is therefore of considerable appeal to patients. As a consequence, anaesthetists are increasingly likely to be asked to deal with patients undergoing this type of surgery.

Advanced laparoscopic surgery presents special problems to the anaesthetist, and may be categorised in the following way.

1. PROBLEMS RELATED TO THE PATIENT

Risk factors in this type of elective surgery are those associated with pre-operative status and possible associated diseases. Age is usually not a particular problem because most patients are in the age group 35–55 years. As these procedures are more widely offered, however, there is likely to be an increasing complication rate linearly related to age (Tiret et al 1992).

2. PROBLEMS RELATED TO THE TECHNIQUE

These operations may be divided into three phases. In phase I, which may last around 20–30 min, a pneumoperitoneum is induced and the uterus and adnexa are surgically isolated. The second phase lasts around 30 min, during which time the operation is completed vaginally, i.e. the vagina is incised and the uterus/adnexa removed. During the third phase, the pneumoperitoneum is re-established for peritoneal toilet and placing of a drain. The abdomen is then emptied of CO_2, a final check for haemostasis is made by suspending the abdominal wall with the 'C' retractor, then the skin incisions are sutured. This phase normally takes 8–12 min. Potential anaesthetic difficulties vary with each phase of the procedure.

INTRA-ABDOMINAL PRESSURE

During the first and second phases of surgery, the intra-abdominal pressure (IAP) is high as a consequence of the pneumoperitoneum of approximately 12–14 mmHg. The pressure of the pneumoperitoneum is regulated by the insufflation device such that a 'ceiling' pressure of 14 mmHg is not exceeded under normal circumstances. Gas flow through the abdominal cavity is in the range of 4–9 $l.min^{-1}$.

It has been estimated that an IAP of 25 mmHg translates as an increased pressure on abdominal organs in the order of 30 $g.cm^{-2}$, with a diaphragmatic pressure of as much as 50 kg. As a direct consequence, pulmonary compliance is reduced. The pressure–volume curve is therefore shifted to the right and its slope is decreased (Fig. 4.1). Although the peak expiratory flow rate (PEFR), forced expiratory volume (FEV) and forced vital capacity (FVC) have been shown to fall significantly after laparoscopic cholecystectomy as a result of the prolonged pneumoperitoneum (tending to return to normal after 24 h, Cooney et al 1992), values for laparoscopic hysterectomy and oophorectomy have yet to be determined.

An IAP of 15 mmHg maintained for 30 min or more is associated with an increase in heart rate and systolic blood pressure (Reid et al 1992). The stroke volume index and cardiac output fall initially, but gradually increase with time. This initial fall is related to a reduction in end-diastolic ventricular index, which occurs as a result of diminished venous return. This is manifest as a transient fall in systemic blood pressure.

The insufflation gas is carbon dioxide, and significant quantities may be absorbed into the systemic circulation across the abdominal peritoneum. Although it is usually possible to maintain a steady end-tidal partial pressure of carbon dioxide, if the intra-abdominal pressure is allowed to rise above 14 mmHg, an increasing rise in end-tidal carbon dioxide partial pressure may be noted which is difficult to rectify (Fig. 4.2). In the absence of other adverse factors, such a marginal rise is harmless.

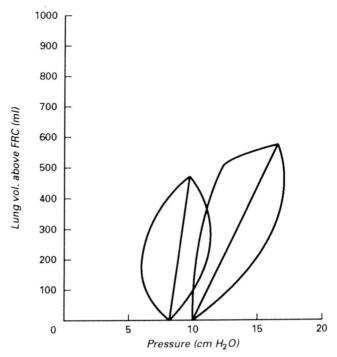

Fig. 4.1 **Pressure–volume curves illustrating changes in lung compliance. FRC, functional residual capacity.**

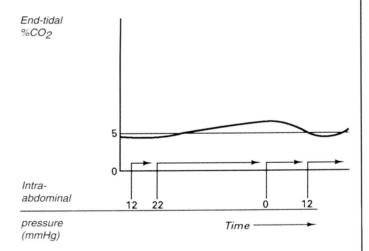

Fig. 4.2 **Capnometer trace showing a slow rise in end-tidal P_{CO_2} in the presence of a high intra-abdominal pressure. %CO_2 falls when the pneumoperitoneum is released but starts rising again when the abdomen is reinsufflated.**

Finally, postoperative nausea has been attributed to abdominal distension, but the relative contribution of the anaesthetic technique per se is difficult to estimate.

POSTURE

The preferred surgical position for these techniques is modified lithotomy (Trendelenburg) with a considerable degree of 'head-down tilt' and the patient's buttocks overhanging the end of the operating table (Fig. 4.3). This is necessary for optimal viewing inside the abdomen during phases I and II of the procedure, since gut may otherwise obscure the operative site. This prolonged posture maintained on the unyielding surface of the operating table may lead to significant backache which may persist for several days. Positioning of the patient's legs is critical, since incorrect positioning may lead to peroneal nerve injury where the inner aspect of the lower leg rests on the lithotomy poles.

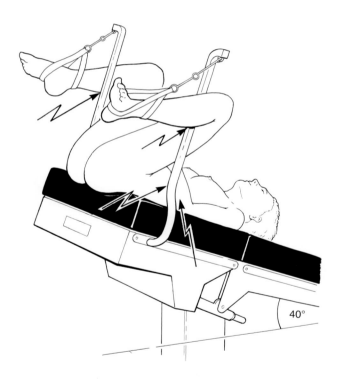

Fig. 4.3 **Steep Trendelenburg position required for laparoscopic surgery. Note high risk areas marked for peripheral diathermy burns – good insulation is mandatory (arrows).**

It is most important to guard the patient's eyes (by taping) because of the risk of either direct trauma from the surgeon (who is often standing close to the patient's head) or from accidents arising from the use of rather long (diathermy-armed) laparoscopic instruments.

THE UNEMPTY STOMACH

60% of patients routinely prepared for surgery have gastric fluid volumes in excess of 40 ml, with a pH of less than 2.5 (Hester et al 1977). This poses a significant problem in many areas of anaesthesia because of the risk of inspiration of gastric contents and Mendelson's syndrome. Of equal concern is the presence of gases inside the stomach. These may be present from the pre-operative phase, but are more likely to result from artificial ventilation using a face mask at the time of induction of anaesthesia. The presence of significant quantities of gas inside the stomach causes a rise in intragastric pressure beyond tolerance of the oesophago-gastric sphincter, thereby increasing the risk of regurgitation and aspiration. The risk of regurgitation is greatest during phases I and III of surgery, when the IAP is maximal and the patient may be in a position of around 40° of 'head-down tilt'.

DURATION OF THE PROCEDURE

Minimally invasive procedures almost invariably require a longer anaesthetic than their 'open' counterpart. More drugs are therefore administered, increasing the potential for manifestation of side effects, and the risks attendant on venous stasis are increased. In general, for operations lasting 30 min or more, there is a linear increase in the complication rate with time (Tiret et al 1986). Autonomic stimulation may lead to irregularities of cardiac rhythm and eventually to cardiac arrest. Cardiac arrest has been attributed to overdistension of the peritoneal cavity during laparoscopy (Arthure 1970). Cardiac arrhythmias, especially severe bradycardia, may occur when the peritoneum is stretched as traction is applied to viscera, although this is, of course, no different to the situation which exists during 'open' hysterectomy.

MISPLACEMENT OF CARBON DIOXIDE

Carbon dioxide pneumothorax has been described as a complication of laparoscopic surgery (Gabbot et al 1992), and may occur following surgical injury to the diaphragm (unlikely in gynaecological surgery), congenital pleuro-peritoneal track or when gas tracks along a subperitoneal route into the pleura. It is more likely to occur when the patient is in steep reverse Trendelenburg position (occasionally required by the surgeon to remove any blood/lavage fluid from the upper abdomen which is there as a result of prolonged 'head-down' positioning). Pneumopericardium and pneumomediastinum (Barker et al 1992) have both been described as complications of laparoscopic surgery, but are exceedingly rare and are highly unlikely to result from gynaecological surgery. Surgical emphysema is very common, but normally insignificant. In extreme cases it may begin to track cephalad, as far as the neck, but in our experience has never led to airway compromise.

Carbon dioxide embolism is a rare but often fatal complication of laparoscopy which usually occurs at the beginning of establishing the pneumoperitoneum due to inadvertent injection of carbon dioxide intravenously via the Verres needle or trochar/cannula (see Chapter 7).

BLOOD LOSS

Blood loss is usually minimal, amounting to less than 300 ml peroperatively with a further 150 ml during the first 24 h postoperatively during uncomplicated procedures. Occasionally, however, if surgical difficulty arises, blood loss may be brisk, and at least two units of blood should be cross-matched for each procedure. Blood transfusion is rarely necessary.

PRE-OPERATIVE MANAGEMENT

This comprises patient assessment, consideration of prophylaxis against thromboembolic disease and prophylactic antibiotic treatment. Pre-operative assessment may be conducted in an outpatient assessment clinic, or alternatively on the day of admission to hospital, provided satisfactory arrangements can be made for any investigations required.

Most women undergoing laparoscopic hysterectomy or oophorectomy are mobile on the first postoperative day and will normally leave hospital on the second or third day. The risk of deep vein thrombosis (DVT) is therefore less than 10% (Salzman & Hirsh 1982), and it is not usually necessary to administer anticoagulants throughout their hospital stay. Prophylactic subcutaneous heparin should be considered in those patients with the following risk factors:

a. age 40 and above
b. established diagnosis of malignancy
c. past history of thromboembolic disorder
d. known thrombocytosis
e. postoperative immobility.

Compression stockings should be used routinely and patients must be kept well hydrated throughout the postoperative period.

We have yet to conduct a prospective randomised trial, but it seems prudent to give all patients prophylactic antibiotics, in view of the prolonged period of communication between the vagina and peritoneal cavity during laparoscopic hysterectomy in particular. Currently we are using cefuroxime 750 mg plus metronidazole 500 mg intravenously at induction.

ANAESTHETIC TECHNIQUE

Airway maintenance

In order to avoid filling the stomach with anaesthetic gases via the face mask, it is prudent to avoid artificial ventilation at induction if it is safe to do so. Pre-oxygenation prior to induction will avoid hypoxaemia and haemoglobin desaturation. The laryngeal mask airway (LMA) is eminently suitable for airway maintenance in this type of surgery, provided airway pressures are not excessive. Leakage of gas does occur during LMA use, but it has been shown that there is no difference in environmental pollution between LMA and endotracheal tube use (Barnett et al 1992). Leakage of inspired gases leads to a discrepancy between the set tidal volume and the delivered tidal volume. The relationship between set tidal volume, expired tidal volume and peak insufflation pressure is illustrated in Figure 4.4. The risk of inhalational pneumonitis with the LMA is not as great in gynaecological laparoscopic surgery as it is in upper abdominal surgery. Surgery on the biliary tract is associated with the secretion of large volumes of gastric juice during the procedure, and the LMA is therefore not recommended for this application. The incidence of regurgitation may be in the order of 25% for the LMA (Barker et al 1992) but there is no evidence that aspiration necessarily occurs in this situation.

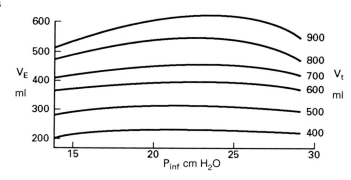

Fig. 4.4 **Effect of inflation pressure (P_{inf}) on expired tidal volume (V_E) for set inspired volume (V_t) using the LMA.**

MUSCLE RELAXATION

Relaxation of the abdominal musculature is necessary, and spontaneous muscular activity which may lead to gagging, coughing and hiccoughing must be avoided. The risk of visceral injury by laparoscopic instruments inside the abdomen is considerable if the patient moves unexpectedly. Return of muscle power before the end of the operation with the patient in lithotomy with a steep 'head-down' position significantly increases the risk of regurgitation of gastric contents and inhalational pneumonitis. It is therefore vital that muscle relaxation is maintained fully until the operation is concluded.

ANAESTHETIC DRUGS

A plan of the overall anaesthetic technique is made at the pre-operative visit. Most patients will require premedication with an anxiolytic (e.g. temazepam 20 mg orally) and an antiemetic agent (e.g. metoclopramide 10 mg orally). If the laryngeal mask is to be used rather than an endotracheal tube, it is important to ensure that the stomach is empty, and therefore the premedication should be given parenterally. An intramuscular combination such as morphine (10 mg), metoclopramide (10 mg) and an H_2 histamine antagonist such as ranitidine (50 mg) provides both patient satisfaction and good working conditions.

Routine monitoring facilities should be established in the anaesthetic room and intravenous access gained under local anaesthesia prior to induction. The combination of cardiostable anaesthetic agents and manipulation of the pelvic viscera can occasionally lead to severe bradycardia. It is therefore advisable to use a prophylactic anticholinergic drug intravenously if none has been given at premedication. Glycopyrrolate 0.2 mg normally suffices to prevent subsequent parasympathetic cardiac effects, but it is prudent to have a further dose ready to administer should the need arise.

Any common induction agent such as thiopentone or etomidate may be used, but the author's preference is propofol (ICI, UK) because induction is less unpleasant than with other agents and the metabolism of the drug is more rapid. This is often strikingly manifest as very good clarity of mind on the first postoperative day. Prilocaine or other local anaesthetic may be used mixed in with the propofol to minimise injection pain, which may occasionally cause distress.

Muscular relaxation may be achieved in the anaesthetic room with any of the available muscle relaxants, but it is not essential at this stage if the LMA is employed; the latter may be inserted and the patient allowed to breathe spontaneously until transfer to the operating room. Muscle relaxation may be achieved by either intermittent bolus injection or continuous infusion according to the anaesthetist's preference.

An anaesthetic vapour in combination with nitrous oxide may be used for maintenance, although a total intravenous anaesthetic is equally suitable. Nitrous oxide is an excellent analgesic (50% nitrous oxide is generally accepted as bioequivalent to 10 mg of morphine) and also acts as a vehicle for anaesthetic vapours mixed with oxygen. Unfortunately, it is highly soluble and therefore crosses semipermeable membranes until the partial pressure is equal on both sides. Gas will thus escape from the blood into gas-containing body cavities such as the digestive tract and peritoneal cavity. Distended bowel or a pneumothorax is therefore likely to worsen in the presence of nitrous oxide. In spite of this, it may safely be used during laparoscopic techniques. It does not lead to bowel distension in operations lasting around 1.5 h (Taylor et al 1992). It does not increase the incidence of postoperative nausea and vomiting.

A typical regime used in the minimally invasive surgery unit is:

Premedication	morphine 10 mg i.m.
	prochlorperazine 12.5 mg i.m.
	ranitidine 50 mg i.m.
	heparin 5000 IU subcutaneously
Induction	glycopyrrolate 0.2 mg i.v.
	propofol 3–5 mg.kg^{-1} i.v.
	atracurium 0.5 mg.kg^{-1} i.v.
	antibiotics: metronidazole 500 mg i.v.
	cefuroxime 750 mg i.v.
	nitrous oxide
	oxygen
	isoflurane
Maintenance	nitrous oxide
	oxygen
	atracurium
	morphine
Postoperative	oxygen
	morphine
	prochlorperazine
	heparin if indicated

MONITORING

Close vigilance must be exercised at all stages, and close contact with the patient must be maintained throughout the duration of the anaesthetic. Such continuous clinical assessment requires supplementation by special monitoring. Monitoring of heart rate and rhythm by electrocardiography is essential throughout the procedure. This allows rapid diagnosis of autonomic activity as well as complications such as pneumothorax. Systemic blood pressure measurement at regular intervals by a non-invasive method will monitor cardiovascular performance in the presence of autonomic stimulation and pneumoperitoneum. Haemorrhage is usually obvious intra-operatively because it is revealed by laparoscopy. It must be borne in mind that the laparoscope magnifies minor bleeding, creating unnecessary anxiety in the unwary.

A pulse oximeter should be used continuously from the time of induction to ensure that haemoglobin desaturation does not occur. This is of particular importance since artificial ventilation using a face mask for preoxygenation is avoided.

A nerve stimulator is essential in helping to assess the degree of muscle relaxation. In its absence it is imperative to administer bolus doses of muscle relaxant at regular intervals or to infuse the drug continuously to avoid loss of relaxation and the attendant complications. Sudden unexpected movements of the patient due to inadequate muscle relaxation (especially hiccoughing) may result in surgical accident if the surgeon is operating close to vital structures.

End-tidal carbon dioxide should be continuously measured using a capnometer which gives a visual display of the four respiratory cycle phases (baseline inspiration, expiration, expiratory pause, inspiration) and is therefore useful for the immediate detection of catastrophic complications such as cardiac arrest, gas embolism or pneumothorax.

POSTOPERATIVE MANAGEMENT

FLUID AND ELECTROLYTE THERAPY
Anaesthetic complications after laparoscopy are in the order of 0.14% (Chamberlain & Brown 1978).

In the absence of high-risk factors for thromboembolic disease it is not necessary to use dextrans. Following a period of pre-operative starvation and dehydration an intravenous regime of 15 ml.kg^{-1}.h^{-1} of crystalloid should be standard during the operation. In addition intra-operative blood loss should be replaced by an appropriate fluid. During the first 24 h postoperatively, a regime of around 1.5–2.0 ml.kg^{-1}.h^{-1} suffices. The regime should include 1.5–2.0 mmol.kg^{-1} bodyweight per day of sodium. It is not normally necessary to administer potassium during the first 24 h but, should an intravenous infusion be necessary beyond this period, 0.5–1.0 mmol.kg^{-1} bodyweight per day should be given to maintain normokalaemia. Early oral fluid intake is encouraged on the first postoperative day and in many cases may be started sooner.

PAIN CONTROL
In uncomplicated cases significant abdominal pain tends to be short-lived (≤24 h) but, if it persists, may herald a surgical complication. Routine methods of postoperative pain relief may be used, although patient-controlled analgesia systems are ideal. From the second day onwards pain is minimal and requires no more than simple analgesics with the possible addition of anti-inflammatory agents. Shoulder-tip pain occurs because of diaphragmatic irritation during the pneumoperitoneum phase of surgery, and minor degrees of small bowel colic are also relatively common. Both tend to settle in 12–36 h. Headache, muscle pain, backache and sore throat are common but short-lived complaints and may be due to both anaesthetic and surgical techniques. Nausea, vomiting and shivering may also occur and may be dealt with using standard therapy.

Urinary retention is very uncommon but must be distinguished from anuria due to urinary tract injury by urethral catheterisation. Light haematuria is common after ureteric catheterisation (during ureteric 'guarding' with stents), but clears rapidly in the presence of good urine flow.

5

LAPAROSCOPIC HYSTERECTOMY: TECHNIQUE

Laparoscopic hysterectomy without bilateral salpingo-oophorectomy

Laparoscopic hysterectomy with bilateral salpingo-oophorectomy

The surgical techniques described for both hysterectomy and oophorectomy involve the use exclusively of endoscopic stapling. Alternative methods of securing haemostasis are endoscopic suturing and bipolar diathermy, as mentioned. Both are perfectly viable techniques, but are more time-consuming and suffer certain drawbacks which have already been alluded to.

LAPAROSCOPIC HYSTERECTOMY WITHOUT BILATERAL SALPINGO-OOPHORECTOMY

It is the opinion of the author that this operation is only justified in those relatively less common cases where very poor vaginal access coexisting with little or no prolapse would make simple vaginal hysterectomy difficult. This operation should be performed relatively uncommonly, since it probably carries little advantage over simple vaginal hysterectomy and is much more expensive both in terms of equipment and theatre time. Claims that patients recover from a laparoscopically assisted procedure faster than from a simple, uncomplicated vaginal hysterectomy have yet to be substantiated. It is conceivable that any advantage seen may be largely due to suggestion (on the part of the surgeon) and psychological (on the part of the patient). A patient who is told that she is undergoing state-of-the-art surgery is more likely to recover rapidly if she is told that she will do so, compared to a patient undergoing an 'old-fashioned' procedure. Conjecture that avoidance of tissue 'bunching' by using staples, and the placing of laparoscopic drains after the procedure, lead to less tissue injury, reduced inflammation and therefore a shorter recovery period has yet to be properly investigated and proved.

However, in the experience of the author, this is a useful operation, although by far the more common application of the technique is when simultaneous oophorectomy is indicated. The technique described in the following section on laparoscopic hysterectomy with bilateral salpingo-oophorectomy is identical to that employed for hysterectomy alone, except that the initial staples are placed medial to the ovaries rather than lateral. Dissection is otherwise the same.

It is worth mentioning that, since the indication for laparoscopic surgery when the ovaries are to be conserved is poor access and descent, special care must be exercised when clamping the uterine artery pedicles. The use of the straight, non-toothed longitudinally ridged forceps already described is essential. These allow gentle and accurate clamping of the tissues without exercising traction on the uterus. At this stage the upper pedicles have already been divided. The risk of shearing of vessels and loss of haemostasis is thus high, and may be very difficult to correct.

Finally, at the time of writing, subtotal laparoscopic hysterectomy is currently under development (K. Semm, personal communication). This technique involves 'coring out' the lower uterus and cervical canal using a transcervical boring tool, followed by a supracervical hysterectomy performed laparoscopically. The substance of the cervix is thus preserved, obviating the need to operate in the vicinity of the ureters and the lower branches of the uterine artery. The superior cervical stump is secured with surgical loops and the superior pedicles with endoscopic sutures. The uterine body is morcellated and extracted via one of the abdominal ports.

At the present time, the future role of this technique is uncertain. It is said that preservation of the cervical 'body' is advantageous in terms of preservation of orgasmic sexual function, although this has not been objectively demonstrated. This theoretical advantage must be balanced against the prophylactic value of cervicectomy against malignancy. Advocates of the procedure contend that since the boring tool 'cores out' the cervix, the possibility of future malignant transformation does not exist, however.

The technique ('CASH') has yet to be widely employed; potential complications (especially those associated with passing a large-diameter cutting tool through the substance of the uterus close to the uterine arteries) have yet to be evaluated. Given the present developed state of the laparoscopic approach with vaginal delivery of the uterus, careful evaluation of yet another new technique will be required.

LAPAROSCOPIC HYSTERECTOMY WITH BILATERAL SALPINGO-OOPHORECTOMY

The following technique includes the laparoscopic division of the uterine arteries. If vaginal access is reasonable, it is possible to include uterine artery dissection in the vaginal part of the operation, and this saves on staple cartridges, which are expensive. However, including the uterine arteries in the laparoscopic dissection, with practice, makes for an overall easier operation. Laparoscopic division of the uterine arteries is to be preferred when vaginal access is limited.

It is strongly recommended that for those embarking upon the technique that ureteric stents are used routinely at first in those cases where the uterine artery is dealt with laparoscopically. The position and proximity of the ureter to the operative site will sometimes surprise even the most experienced of endoscopic surgeons and the most knowledgeable of anatomists. A sobering exercise is to place the stapler jaws over the uterine artery pedicle after bladder dissection, where it is *thought* that the ureter is clear, then to activate the transilluminating ureteric stent. The true position of the ureter is sometimes unanticipated.

The standard technique we are currently employing is as follows:

A 10 mm trochar and cannula is inserted beneath the umbilicus to allow passage of the 10 mm laparoscope. Pre-insufflation using a Verres needle is still favoured by some surgeons, but direct entry into the abdomen with the 10 mm trochar and cannula is probably equally safe and possibly safer, especially if the self-guarding disposable type is used. The disadvantage of using a Verres needle is that it is a small-diameter, relatively sharp device, and hence easily capable of penetrating structures inside the abdomen, despite the sprung guard. If the guard spring is compressed by the pressure of the layers of the abdominal wall as it enters the abdomen, why should it not be compressed if the distal end of the needle strikes other structures, thus revealing the sharp end of the needle itself? Moreover, inadvertent entry into large blood vessels, especially veins whose low pressure may mean that injury is *not* declared by a tell-tale rush of blood from the operator end, may result in intravascular carbon dioxide injection and potentially fatal gas embolism. Finally, checking if the end of the needle lies in the peritoneal cavity by placing a drop of saline on the end of the needle to see if it disappears, is pointless. The drop of saline will still disappear if the end of the needle lies within bowel lumen, or even if it lies within the lumen of the vena cava, whose contents may often be at negative pressure. Many surgeons are now abandoning the Verres needle.

The laparoscope should be clean and dry, with the eyepiece (unless the telescope and camera are a single integrated unit) meticulously cleaned and dried prior to camera attachment. Unless the surgeon has access to a purpose-designed telescope warming device (these are available, but are exceedingly expensive and unnecessary), the distal end of the telescope should be immersed for at least 2 min in sterile water which is at least 45°C. This 2 min is time well spent and will obviate the need to repeatedly wipe the end of the telescope because of misting.

The abdomen is insufflated using a high-flow insufflator unit. Two 12 mm trochar and cannulae are passed into the abdominal cavity under direct vision, 150 mm apart either side of the midline just above the pubis (Fig. 5.1). The inferior epigastric vessels are avoided either by transilluminating the puncture sites prior to incision or by direct laparoscopic inspection of the interior abdominal wall. An assistant cannulates the cervix using a Spackman cannula and vulsellum forceps to allow vaginal manipulation of the uterus and adnexa. The 12 mm ports may be fitted as required with reducing adaptors to allow the passage of 5 mm instruments without loss of gas.

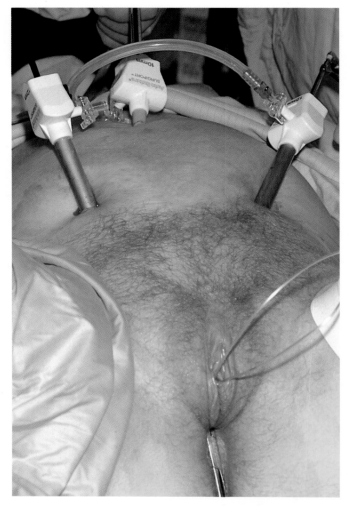

Fig. 5.1 **Positioning of cannulae. Note transilluminating ureteric stents.**

The uterus is then deviated by the assistant to the contralateral side to the initial operative site to allow maximum access. The ovarian ligament is grasped using self-locking laparoscopic forceps via the lower cannula on the opposite side to the initial operating site, and the ovary and tube placed 'on stretch' to expose the infundibulopelvic ligament (Fig. 5.2). The Endo Gauge™ is inserted through the cannula on the operations side and the tissue thickness of the infundibulopelvic ligament is measured. This almost invariably indicates that a 3.5 mm cartridge (blue coded) is required.

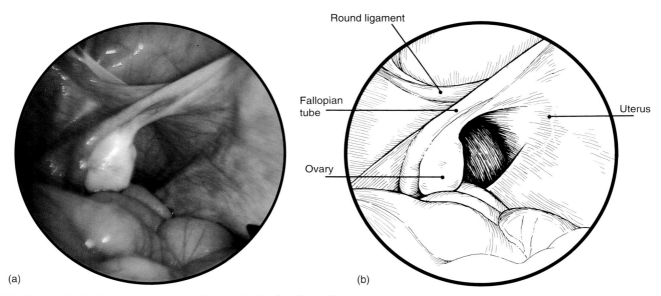

(a)   (b)

Fig. 5.2 **Exposed left adnexa – suitable uterine angulation for dissection.**

The Multifire Endo GIA™ stapler then replaces the Endo Gauge™. The jaws may be closed over the infundibulopelvic and round ligaments simultaneously or, if this proves to be an excessive amount of tissue, the infundibulopelvic ligament alone (Fig. 5.3a and b).

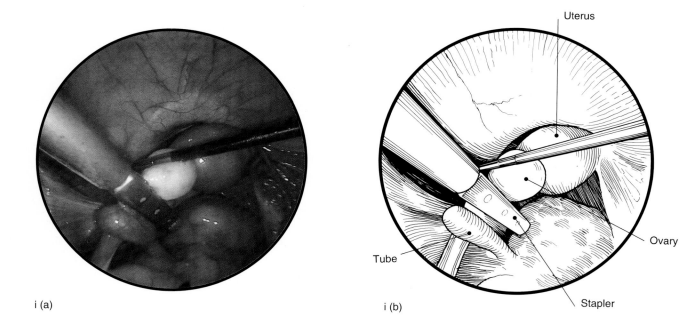

i (a) i (b)

Fig. 5.3 **Multifire Endo GIA**™ **stapler applied to left infundibulopelvic ligament (a), and appearance after firing (b).**

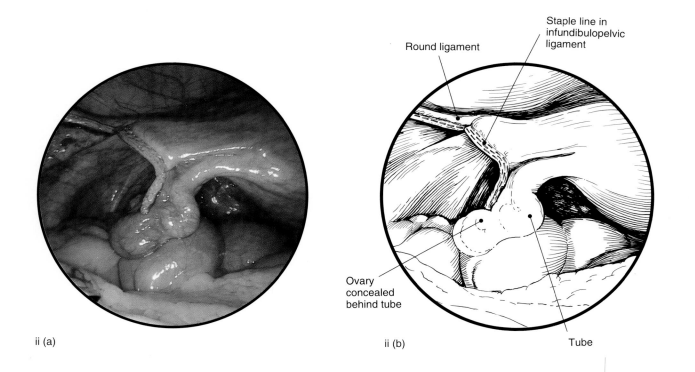

ii (a) ii (b)

The actuating lever which clamps the stapler jaws should be easily moved into the closed position. If there is resistance to closure, excessive tissue has been loaded into the jaws. The most common reason for this is that the tip of one pole of the ovary has been inadvertently clamped. The lever should never be *forced* to close; this invariably results in loss of haemostasis and failure to divide tissues. Since the jaws of the instrument are rotatable, optimal application geometry may be achieved with a simultaneous comfortable hand-position.

At this stage it is vital to thoroughly examine the tissues clamped. The distal tip of the stapler must be in the 'clear' area of the broad ligament to avoid partial transection of vessels and failure of haemostasis. Care must be taken to avoid the bladder edge and 'tenting' of the pelvic side wall peritoneum to exclude the possibility of damage to the bladder or ureter. In our experience, there is rarely need to dissect the round and infundibulopelvic ligaments separately. If, however, the round ligament is excluded from this first stapling, it may be included in the diathermy/scissors dissection for the bladder. Ensuring that the tip of the stapler does not extend below the 'bare area' of the broad ligament, and that the jaws of the instrument are closed immediately lateral to the ovary (i.e. as far from the pelvic side-wall as possible), ensures that the ureter is clear of the operative site.

In difficult cases, or where there is concern about the position of the ureters, transilluminating stents (Uriglow™, Rocket of London Ltd, Watford, UK; Fig. 5.4) may be placed cystoscopically, which means that the ureter is easily identified as a row of glowing points (Fig. 5.5). A 30° operating cystoscope with an operating channel at least 2 mm in diameter should be used. The stents should be handled with care to avoid kinking and damage to the fibreoptic strands which may cause 'spillage' of light from cracks and thus a loss in light intensity inside the ureter. It is important that the stents are lubricated with sterile, water-soluble jelly to facilitate easy insertion and minimise trauma to the ureters. The stents are graduated with blue lines at 10 mm intervals so that depth of insertion may be judged. There is also a red marker which should lie at or close to the urethral meatus, allowing accurate placement. 'Fine tuning' of the stent position may be accomplished under laparoscopic control. Under no circumstance should the stent be advanced too far to avoid the theoretical possibility of traumatising the renal calyces. Occasionally, light haematuria may be noted for a few hours postoperatively, but this may be avoided by gentle insertion and keeping stent movement to a minimum once they are in situ.

Although the stents may not be visualised within the ureteric canal (where they are most vulnerable to injury), the exclusion of the ureter from the stapler may be verified as follows: at the medial point at which the ureter 'disappears' into the ureteric canal, its course runs directly anteriorly and inferiorly. Placing of the tip of the stapler medial to the point of disappearance means that the ureter *cannot* be trapped. Secondly, once the stapler jaws are closed, but *not* fired, the stent on that side should be agitated back and forth by a few millimetres. Free transmission of that movement (seen by movement of the glowing stent in the ureter as it lies parallel to the uterosacral ligament) makes doubly certain that the ureter is not injured.

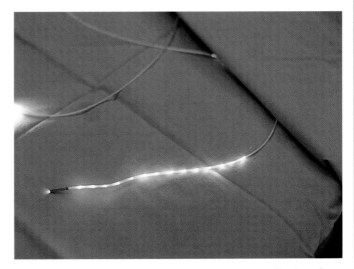

Fig. 5.4 **Uriglow™ transilluminating ureteric stents** (Rocket of London Ltd).

43

When the surgeon is satisfied that the stapler is placed correctly, it may then be 'fired'. It is essential that the jaws remain in the clamped position for a minimum of 1 min prior to firing to allow the entrapped tissues to be compressed and tissue fluid expressed. This ensures good staple fixation and therefore haemostasis. Adequate tissue compression may be judged when the tissues either side of the jaws of the stapler appear whitish and devascularised. Once again, the stapler jaws should not be excessively loaded with tissue. Premature firing of the stapler may lead to loss of haemostasis. The process is repeated on the opposite side.

Using a non-self-locking forceps and scissors, the bladder is then freed from the anterior wall of the uterus, uniting the inferior ends of the incisions achieved with the stapler (Fig. 5.6). Bladder dissection then proceeds until the vaginal wall is reached (Fig. 5.7). This may be verified by the assistant placing a finger in the anterior fornix – the vagina, stripped free from bladder, is easily identified by the surgeon. It is important at this stage not to incise the vaginal wall because of loss of pneumoperitoneum.

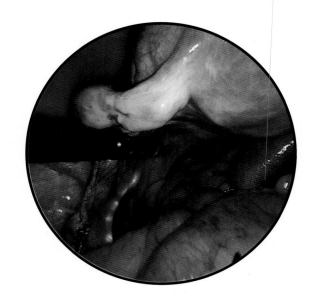

Fig. 5.5 **Transilluminating stent in situ.**

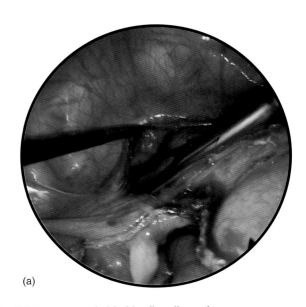

(a)

Fig. 5.6 **Laparoscopic bladder flap dissection.**

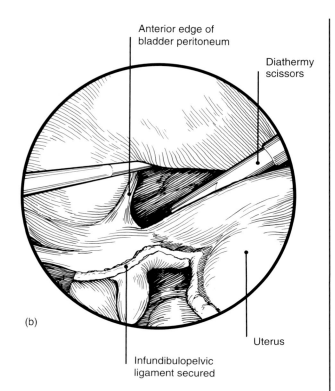

(b)

Anterior edge of
bladder peritoneum

Diathermy
scissors

Uterus

Infundibulopelvic
ligament secured

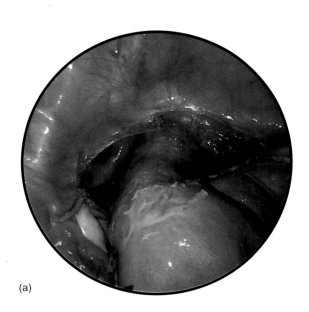

(a)

Fig. 5.7 **Completed bladder flap dissection. Note appearance of cervix.**

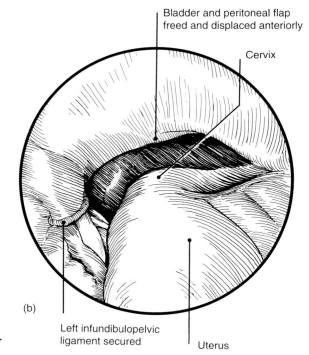

(b)

Bladder and peritoneal flap
freed and displaced anteriorly

Cervix

Left infundibulopelvic
ligament secured

Uterus

Working again laterally, the lateral margins of the freed bladder must be identified, and the surgeon must be satisfied that the uterine arteries are exposed. The stapler is then re-introduced and the uterine arteries are clamped and divided (Fig. 5.8). The surgeon must carefully examine the tissue included in the clamp before the stapler is fired to preclude the possibility of damage to the bladder or ureters. Occasionally, a small vessel in the inferior margin of the uterine artery pedicle may fail to be controlled by the stapler and may need to be sealed with diathermy.

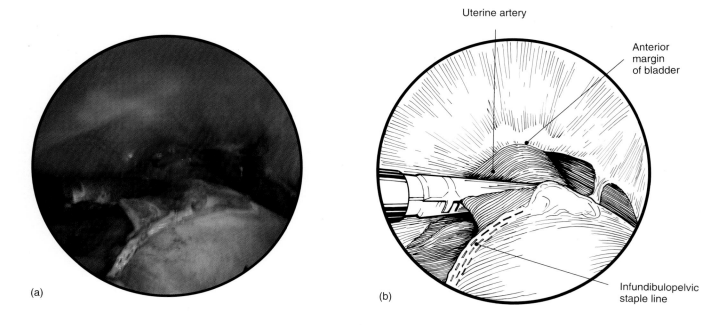

(a)

(b)

Uterine artery

Anterior margin of bladder

Infundibulopelvic staple line

Fig. 5.8 **Multifire Endo GIA™ stapler applied to left uterine artery pedicle.**

At this stage, the laparoscopic dissection is complete. Although it is possible to divide the uterosacral ligaments and divide the vagina from the cervix circumferentially via the laparoscope, this is more easily achieved vaginally. Moreover, completing the operation vaginally obviates the need to use further endoscopic staples or suturing techniques, reducing operative time and cost.

The laparoscopic ports should be left in situ to allow inspection of the uterine bed at the end of the procedure to ensure haemostasis, perform peritoneal toilet with a wash/suction device, and to place a vacuum drain in situ.

The vaginal dissection may then be started. It is worth mentioning again that it is *essential* that the surgeon's assistant(s) are aware of the special need for avoiding excessive traction when completing this phase of the operation. Without the support of the round and infundibulopelvic ligaments, the smaller branches of the uterine artery are easily sheared off from the lateral aspect of the body of the uterus, leading to loss of haemostasis which, as mentioned, may be very difficult indeed to control. This is by far the most common cause of bleeding. If ureteric stents have been placed in situ to protect the ureters, they should remain in place until the vaginal dissection is finished. The reason for this is that if haemostasis is not secure by the time the uterus is completely removed, and extra sutures are needed to control bleeding from the uterine artery pedicles, it is not impossible to damage or obstruct the ureter at this stage.

The cervix is grasped using two pairs of vulsellum forceps and the dissection proceeds much as for vaginal hysterectomy, although certain aspects require emphasis. The pouch of Douglas is opened using a knife to incise the posterior fornix vaginal skin and peritoneum. At this stage, the surgeon will be aware of whether or not the abdomen has been fully depressurised; if it has not, the peritoneum will bulge outwards. Although this makes identification of the peritoneum easier, the remainder of the carbon dioxide should be drained via one of the cannulae before proceeding, because of the risk of pressurised blood and peritoneal fluid being sprayed into the surgeon's face.

Once access is gained to the peritoneal cavity, the uterosacral ligaments may then be clamped, divided and ligated using angulated clamps or aneurysm needles in the usual way. Circumcision of the cervix is then completed circumferentially and the uterovesical pouch is opened to unite with the laparoscopic bladder dissection. Once entry is gained to the peritoneal cavity both anteriorly and posteriorly, the bladder (and therefore the ureters) should be swept digitally laterally and superiorly to ensure that the urinary tract is clear of the operative field. If ureteric stents have been used, the ureters may be easily palpated and avoided.

At this stage, if the uterine artery pedicle has not been dealt with laparoscopically, the tissue remaining to be divided consists of the whole of the uterine artery pedicle, bearing both the artery itself and its small branches, up to the 'bare area' of the broad ligament (Fig. 5.9). If the uterine artery has been dealt with laparoscopically, there remains only a small pedicle connecting the uterus to the parametrium, which must, however, be formally clamped, divided and ligated. This small volume of tissue often contains small branches of the uterine artery which have not been controlled laparoscopically. The remaining tissue may then be clamped, divided and ligated.

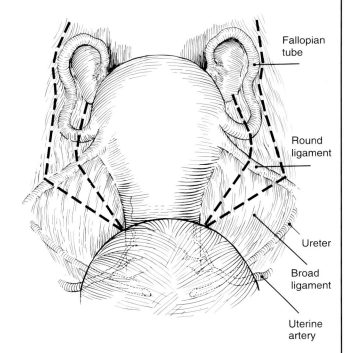

Fallopian tube

Round ligament

Ureter

Broad ligament

Uterine artery

Fig. 5.9 **Dissection at conclusion of laparoscopic dissection – uterine arteries are shown undivided.**

Whichever method has been used to control the uterine artery, it is important that the surgeon feels both anteriorly and posteriorly for the inferior margin of the laparoscopic dissection. This is best achieved by an exploring finger placed through the posterior fornix, past the (ligated) uterosacral ligaments and anteriorly through the uterovesical pouch. If staples have been used, they are easily detected. Alternatively, the abdominal wall may be suspended in order to maintain vision inside the abdomen, even after desufflation, by using a special 'C' retractor (Rocket of London Ltd; Fig. 5.10). This enables the surgeon to elevate the abdominal wall by inserting the pointed end of the 'C' retractor through one of the 12 mm incisions and sliding the inserted arm transversely on the inside of the abdominal wall, and lifting. The vaginal surgeon may then control placement of the haemostatic clamps under direct vision (Fig. 5.11).

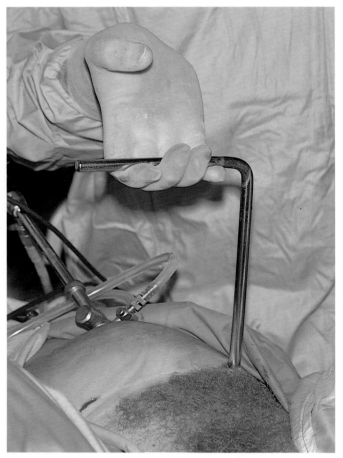

Fig. 5.10 **C-shaped abdominal wall retractor in situ.**

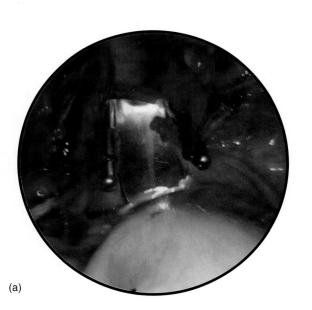

(a)

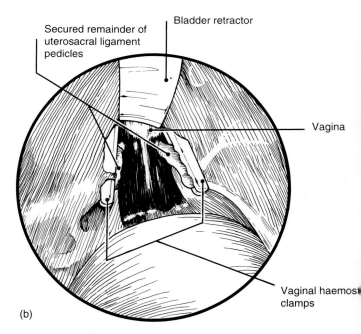

Secured remainder of uterosacral ligament pedicles

Bladder retractor

Vagina

Vaginal haemostatic clamps

(b)

Fig. 5.11 **Laparoscopic view of vaginal clamps completing the uterine artery dissection. The tips of the clamps are clearly demonstrated.**

As mentioned, the author favours the use of straight, non-toothed longitudinally ridged or 'cross-hatched' clamps. These allow tissue clamping by sliding the jaws of the clamp over the remaining pedicle, accompanied by the exploring finger, to ensure that the tip of the clamp meets and includes the inferior margin of the staple line. Failure to include this area inevitably leads to failure of haemostasis. Occasionally, if the uterine arteries have not been dealt with laparoscopically, the remaining tissue is too large in volume to be safely dealt with by a single clamp, and must be dealt with as two pedicles.

The major advantage of laparoscopically dividing the uterine artery pedicle is that only a single application of the vaginal clamp is required. If two applications of the vaginal clamp are required, great care must be exercised to ensure that a 'window' of unsecured tissue does not remain between the two pedicles. This is best achieved by tying the two together after the uterus is removed, to eliminate potential 'dead space'. Similarly, if two pedicles are created, it is important to examine the tissue clamped after the first 'bite' is taken to ensure that a large vessel is not partially clamped and partially free at the tip of the clamp. It is recommended that one side is completed at a time (i.e. clamped, divided and ligated), since there is usually insufficient space for *two* clamps *and* the exploring finger in the uterovesical pouch incision.

Once the uterus has been removed, the uterine bed should then be thoroughly inspected vaginally for bleeding. Sometimes it is possible to visualise the whole of the dissection, including the staples in the infundibulopelvic ligament, but more often the latter requires laparoscopic inspection. If extra sutures are required to secure a leaking pedicle, special care must be taken laterally to avoid the ureters.

It cannot be emphasised too strongly that the temptation to use traction on the uterus during the final stages of its removal to improve access must be resisted at all costs. Even mild traction may lead to problematic bleeding if a small branch of the uterine artery is sheared off flush with the pelvic side wall.

One special circumstance deserves special mention. If the uterus is significantly enlarged by fibroids to the extent that extracting the uterus through the pelvic outlet is likely to prove 'tight', the possibility of 'snagging' the haemostatic staples on the infundibulopelvic and uterine artery pedicles must be borne in mind. The sides of the isolated uterus are of course also studded with staples, which may catch and even avulse those securing the pedicles, leading to potentially severe loss of haemostasis. This may be avoided by rotating the isolated uterus through 90° prior to extraction. The two lines of staples on the uterus and pelvic sidewall are thereby rotationally separated, and snagging avoided.

It is the experience of the author that there is no need to close the peritoneum separately, although it should be included in the vaginal skin stitch to prevent bleeding. The uterosacral ligaments may be united in the usual way by tying them together. Although there is usually no need to use a vaginal pack for haemostasis, packing of the vagina makes subsequent laparoscopic inspection of the uterine bed easier, since it 'tents' the vault and exposes the dissection line. Bladder catheterisation for 24 h enables the patient to rest without getting out of bed, but this must be balanced against the increased risk of urinary tract infection.

The abdomen is re-insufflated and the uterine bed is checked for haemostasis. Insufflation pressure should be kept to a minimum consistent with good visualisation because higher pressures may conceal venous leakage. Any leaking vessel may then be dealt with using bipolar diathermy, although the possible proximity of the ureters must always be kept in mind. It is very important to avoid applying unipolar diathermy to tissue-bearing staples. If current is applied directly to the staple line, the tissue immediately surrounding each staple will necrose, resulting in potential loss of haemostasis. A final check is made in the absence of a pneumoperitoneum using the 'C' abdominal wall retractor.

A small-bore vacuum drain is then placed under direct vision in the uterine bed. The easiest method of achieving this is to 'feed' the drain tube through one of the lower cannulae. If disposable 12 mm cannulae with 5.5 mm reducers have been used, this may be easily accomplished by introducing the distal end of the drain through the reducing plate, opening the gas seal manually via the operating lever on the side of the cannula, inserting the drain fully into place, then removing the cannula from around the drain. The drain tubing may then be secured with sutures. The abdominal puncture sites are closed with 2-0 Dexon or similar dissolving suture.

The drain should be placed under vacuum, and under normal circumstances should not drain more than 200 ml in the first 24 h postoperatively (bearing in mind that some saline wash is invariably left behind in the abdominal cavity following peritoneal toilet). If significantly more blood than this drains during this time period, then failure of haemostasis should be suspected (see Ch. 7).

6

LAPAROSCOPIC OOPHORECTOMY: TECHNIQUE

Simple laparoscopic bilateral oophorectomy where the ovaries are normal (or appear normal) for the adjunctive treatment of breast cancer is a procedure ever more in demand. Removal of ovarian cysts or suspected ovarian malignancies using laparoscopic techniques are outside the scope of this book; there are any number of colour atlases on the broader subject of general gynaecological laparoscopic surgery which deal with this topic adequately.

This chapter deals with the removal of essentially normal ovaries, when the uterus is to remain in situ.

Three-point entry is gained to the abdominal cavity in the usual way, using a single 10 mm trochar and cannula just beneath the umbilicus for the laparoscope, and two 12 mm cannulae either side of the midline just above the pubic hair line, approximately 150 mm apart. Using either the Multifire Endo GIA™ stapler (or bipolar diathermy and scissors, but see discussion above concerning hazards of diathermy), the ovary is isolated and excised using two dissection lines to form a V-shaped 'wedge' of tissue (Fig. 6.1).

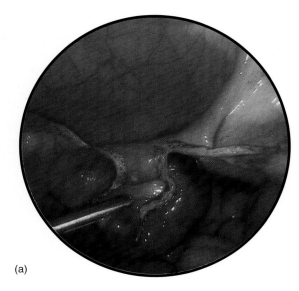

(a)

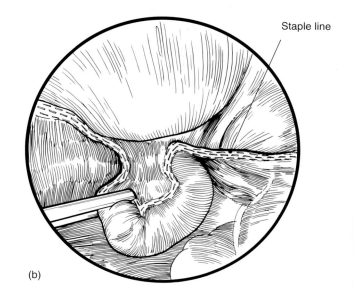

Staple line

(b)

Fig. 6.1 **Right ovary isolated using staples.**

The surgeon is then left with the choice of either removing the ovaries through the abdominal wall or retrieving them from the pouch of Douglas via a posterior colpotomy. The disadvantage of using the abdominal route is that morcellation of some description will be required, unless the ovaries are very small indeed. This makes histological analysis much more difficult, which may be important in cases of possible malignant spread from the breast.

Those who have attempted to simply grasp the ovaries and pull them through the abdominal wall will attest to the potential difficulties of this manoeuvre. It is quite often the case that the ovaries will pass without difficulty through the peritoneum, muscle and fat, but then become trapped either by fascia or by skin. In the relatively obese patient, this can present a very difficult situation to deal with: an ovary 'lost' in the abdominal wall. Oedema and blood may make subsequent retrieval almost impossible without a larger incision.

An easier method of extraction, which, however, suffers the disadvantage that a vaginal incision is required (and therefore a greater risk of infection exists), is to exit via the pouch of Douglas. Antibiotic prophylaxis is mandatory. Once the ovaries are lying free in the abdomen and haemostasis is ensured, the ovaries are then placed under direct vision into a laparoscopic tissue retrieval bag (Figs 6.2 and 6.3; Vernon-Carus Ltd, UK).

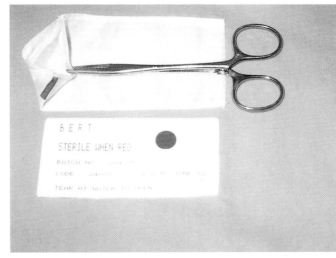

Fig. 6.2 **Endoscopic tissue retrieval bag (Vernon Carus Ltd, UK).**

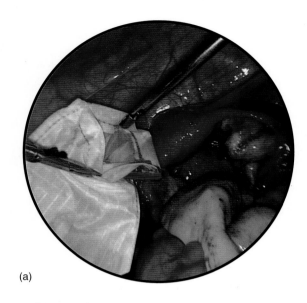

(a)

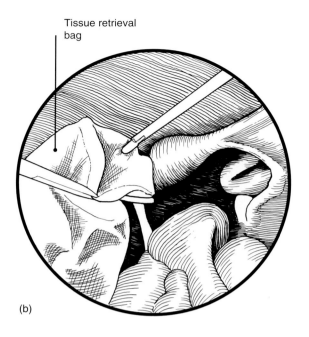

Tissue retrieval bag

(b)

Fig. 6.3 **Tissue retrieval bag in situ.**

The vaginal assistant then makes a small (5 mm) midline incision in the posterior fornix, cutting through the vaginal skin only, leaving the peritoneum intact, thus preserving the pneumo-peritoneum. A heavy snipe-nosed self-locking laparoscopic grasping forceps is then inserted into the vaginal incision and, exercising great care to remain exactly in the midline, gently pushed through the peritoneum while the laparoscopic surgeon monitors the progress of the instrument under direct vision. It is *essential* that the peritoneum is perforated in the midline and that

the forceps is not allowed to 'wander' laterally. This might obviously result in damage to the ureter or the uterine artery, leading to disaster – broad ligament haematoma. Similarly, angulation of the forceps in the vertical plane must be accurate to achieve 'clean' entry into the pouch. If the distal end of the forceps is pushed in too far anteriorly, it is likely that the substance of the uterine body will be penetrated, leading to bleeding. Too far posteriorly means that the rectum is liable to be damaged.

Once the vaginal forceps has entered the peritoneal cavity, the leading edge of the tissue retrieval bag containing the ovaries is 'offered' by the laparoscopic surgeon (using graspers) to the opened jaws of the vaginal forceps (Fig. 6.4). The vaginal surgeon then locks the jaws of his forceps over the leading edge of the retrieval bag and gently draws it into the pouch, causing 'tenting' of the posterior fornix towards him. Using a long-handled knife, the original 5 mm incision is then gradually widened at its lateral margins and the abdomen is simultaneously depressurised (to prevent pressurised blood and peritoneal fluid from contaminating the vaginal surgeon's face). The bag and its contents are then delivered vaginally and the posterior colpotomy is closed with dissolving sutures. The abdomen is re-insufflated, haemostasis is checked and peritoneal toilet is performed. A final check is made without pneumoperitoneum, using the 'C' retractor. A laparoscopically placed drain may be left in situ if there is any persistent 'oozing' (viewed without pneumoperitoneum) but this is only occasionally necessary, in the author's experience. Postoperative recovery time is usually only 24 h.

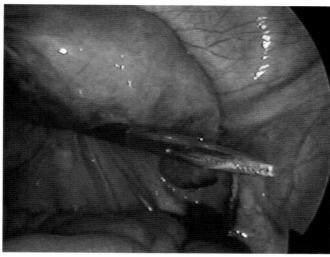

Fig. 6.4 **Laparoscopic forceps inserted transvaginally through posterior fornix.**

7

COMPLICATIONS OF LAPAROSCOPIC SURGERY

M. John

General complications

Specific complications of laparoscopic surgery

Laparoscopic hysterectomy and oophorectomy are relatively new techniques, and little has been written concerning specific complications or incidence of problems. Complications may arise as a direct result of laparoscopy per se or as a consequence of surgical methods peculiar to each technique. The majority of complications associated with laparoscopic hysterectomies can be avoided by careful pre-operative selection of subjects, skilled operative technique and good postoperative care. However, when complications do occur, early recognition and prompt treatment will ensure the best possible outcome.

Hysterectomy is one of the commonest of all major operations and is associated with a significant complication rate. The mortality rate directly attributed to hysterectomy is reported as between 0.05% and 0.2% (Sharp & Jordan 1987). Less easy to assess is the morbidity resulting from complications. In common with most major surgical procedures, infection and haemorrhage are the most frequently encountered problems. Injury to the urinary tract is a hazard more specific to hysterectomy and has been reported to occur in 1.5% of cases (Daly & Higgins 1988). However, vaginal hysterectomy carries a much lower complication rate than abdominal hysterectomy (Sharp & Jordan 1987, Dicker et al 1982).

Laparoscopic total hysterectomy and oophorectomy demands a high level of hand–eye coordination and laparoscopic surgical skills which may not lie immediately within the repertoire of the general gynaecologist. This potential deficit of experience has been recognised and extensive retraining and study advised by some authorities (Garry 1992). Complex gynaecological laparoscopic surgery demands new skills from the whole surgical team – the camera/laparoscope 'operator' (whose job may often be most difficult), the vaginal assistant, scrub-nurse and technician must all be adequately trained and experienced for successful surgery. Surgeons with little or no experience or training in operative laparoscopy 'having a go' may cause a disaster; this practice should be deplored. These procedures should be carried out by suitably trained surgeons with adequate experience who have access to the correct equipment and are familiar with its use. In the future, it may well be that the medico-legal situation in any hospital will enforce untrained practitioners to refrain from incautious attempts at surgery for which they are not trained, by formal censure and legal penalty should complications occur.

GENERAL COMPLICATIONS

Anaesthesia

Anaesthetic technique and complications are discussed in Chapter 4.

The Confidential Enquiry into Gynaecological Laparoscopy of the Royal College of Obstetricians and Gynaecologists (Chamberlain & Brown 1978) identified the following major anaesthetic complications encountered in a review of over 12 000 cases:

1. Bronchospasm, urticaria, hypotension following thiopentone induction
2. General peripheral vasodilatation following althesin
3. Failure or difficulty in intubation
4. Regurgitation of stomach contents at induction
5. Gaseous distension of the stomach at induction
6. Tachycardia (>120 beats/min)
7. Suxamethonium apnoea
8. Incomplete reversal of non-depolarising relaxants
9. Peroperative hypotension/hypertension
10. Tetany (hyperventilation)
11. Postoperative hypotension
12. Coronary insufficiency
13. Laryngospasm at extubation
14. Severe postoperative vomiting
15. Opiate overdose

Many of the anaesthetic problems associated with these procedures are related to gas insufflation and the pneumoperitoneum (Ch. 4).

INFECTION

Postoperative infection following laparoscopic surgery may arise in the abdominal wounds, pelvis, chest or urinary tract. Several studies have demonstrated that the use of prophylactic antibiotics substantially reduces morbidity among women undergoing vaginal hysterectomy (Polk et al 1980, Duff & Park 1980). On this basis, prophylactic antibiotics are advocated for all laparoscopic hysterectomies, although prospective controlled trials (if justified) are awaited. The prolonged surgical communication of the vagina and the peritoneal cavity means that infection with Gram-negative and anaerobic bacteria is especially likely, and antibiotic 'cover' should reflect this. Strict aseptic technique during ureteric catheterisation is especially important because of the risk of ascending urinary tract infection.

THROMBOEMBOLISM

The short period of immobilisation and hospitalisation associated with laparoscopic surgery may be expected to result in lowering the risk of venous thrombosis. However, in high-risk patients the use of antiembolic stockings and prophylactic heparin is prudent. Pelvic haematoma and pelvic abscess increase the likelihood of venous thrombosis and septic pelvic thrombophlebitis, and are possible complications of this type of surgery. Although the place of subcutaneous heparin in these circumstances has yet to be fully clarified, it is recommended that anticoagulant prophylaxis is started as soon as the diagnosis is suspected (5000 IU calcium heparin subcutaneously twice daily). The routine placing of a suction drain at the operation site is an effective method of reducing the risk of haematoma.

SPECIFIC COMPLICATIONS OF LAPAROSCOPIC SURGERY

Penetrating injuries following accessing the peritoneal cavity

Verres needle preinsufflation is not practised in the technique described here. A guarded, disposable 10 mm trochar and cannula (Surgiport™, Auto Suture Company) or a reusable trochar and cannula with the gas inflow tap opened is introduced directly into the peritoneal cavity. The rationale for this 'direct entry' technique is described in Chapter 5.

Direct trauma to bowel, bladder and other pelvic organs is well recognised. Catheterisation and emptying of the bladder and pelvic examination under anaesthesia to exclude an unexpected pelvic mass reduces such risk of injury. Perforation of bowel is more likely when there has been previous abdominal surgery or adhesion formation. Techniques are currently under development where the abdominal cavity is entered under direct vision using transparent-ended trochars (K. Semm, personal communication).

Trochar/cannula insertion technique is extremely important, although it is expected that the reader will have developed his own reliable and safe method. Confining the plane of the trochar on first entry (beneath the umbilicus) to the midline, 45° from horizontal, making certain the point does not 'wander' away from the midline on entering the peritoneal cavity (thus avoiding potential injury to the great vessels) and emplacement of the other two trochar/cannulae only under direct laparoscopic vision are the essential ingredients of safe entry into the peritoneal cavity. Should bowel injury occur, the experienced laparoscopist should recognise the fact: the trochar point is contaminated with bowel contents and the injury may be visible (unless the bowel is tightly adherent to the anterior abdominal wall).

If large vessel injury does occur, above all, it is vital not to withdraw the trochar/cannula. It is routine practice for all junior doctors joining the team to be specifically instructed on this point. Fatal haemorrhage may be avoided by *leaving the cannula with its tip inside the vessel lumen should vascular injury occur*. The abdomen may then be opened and the injury easily identified and repaired by a vascular surgeon. If the cannula is withdrawn, the patient may exsanguinate by the time the abdomen can be opened, or a smaller tear bleed retroperitoneally, making subsequent identification and remedy exceedingly difficult.

GAS INSUFFLATION

Misplacing of carbon dioxide, its consequences and the anaesthetic problems posed by a prolonged, relatively high-pressure pneumoperitoneum are discussed in Chapter 4.

The use of a high-flow insufflator increases the risk of extraperitoneal insufflation and surgical emphysema. Care must be taken to ensure that the cannula bearing the gas supply does not inadvertently slip into the extraperitoneal space. Extraperitoneal insufflation is not a major problem but on occasion may lead to a failed insufflation and abandoning of the procedure or impair visibility.

HAEMORRHAGE

Haemorrhage complicating a laparoscopic hysterectomy may be primary, reactionary or secondary. Meticulous haemostasis must be maintained throughout the procedure as blood in the peritoneal cavity absorbs light, impairing visibility, which may make subsequent attempts to secure faulty haemostasis very difficult indeed. An efficient washer-sucker device is invaluable in dealing with haemorrhage; a warm (approximately 35°C) normal saline solution is ideal for lavage and for disrupting clots. A 5 mm device is usually sufficient, although 10 mm washer/suckers are available. Great care must be taken to avoid suction or avulsion injury to bowel, which easily becomes attached to the instrument. This risk is worse with the 10 mm device. The blood and saline may then be aspirated, although considerable vacuum may be required to manage clot suction (–40 mmHg). The end of the instrument must at all times be 'buried' in the liquid/clot being aspirated, otherwise loss of pneumoperitoneum is very rapid indeed.

Loss of haemostasis due to incorrect or inappropriate staple application is discussed in Chapter 3.

The commonest site of intraoperative haemorrhage is between the uterine artery pedicle which is secured laparoscopically and the utero-sacral and cardinal ligaments which are divided and ligated vaginally. This occurs because the stapler is occasionally fired across the uterine artery pedicle with some of the small inferior branches of the artery 'missed'. These branches are avulsed if downward traction is applied to the uterus – as is customary in a vaginal hysterectomy. These small vessels retract into the loose areolar tissue of the parametrium and the paracolpium. Usually, it is not difficult to ligate these bleeding vessels vaginally, but at the end of the dissection, *it is vital that the inferior end of the laparoscopic dissection line and the superior end of the vaginal dissection line meet*. After the uterus has been removed, the anterior abdominal wall is elevated using the 'C' retractor, introduced through one of the lower abdominal incisions under direct vision while the abdomen is still filled with gas. The operation site can then be inspected for any signs of bleeding without a positive intra-abdominal pressure. Bleeding pedicles may then be dealt with either abdominally or vaginally, according to which route offers the easiest access.

Haemostasis may be achieved by clamping and ligating any leaking vessels vaginally in the conventional manner, if the bleeding point is sufficiently low down. On occasion haemostasis has to be achieved endoscopically and several different techniques are available to arrest bleeding and produce haemostasis. Diathermy electrocoagulation is effective but potentially hazardous (see Ch. 3), although bipolar diathermy forceps are ideal for controlling 'ooze' from a small imperfectly controlled pedicle. Individual endoscopic titanium clips, endoscopic sutures or loops may also be used if the bleeding is arising from pedunculated tissue.

Leakage from tissue which is 'flush' with the pelvic side-wall is especially difficult to control, since there is nothing to affix loops or staples to. Under these circumstances, unipolar diathermy coagulation or emplacing haemostatic sutures using laparoscopic suturing techniques may be effective, but the position of the ureters *must* be defined. This is especially true of the operative site when small branches of the uterine artery pedicle have been inadvertently 'sheared' off because of imprudent traction on the uterus during the vaginal dissection phase of the operation.

Dividing the uterovesical fold of peritoneum and freeing the bladder base from the anterior aspect of the uterus and cervix is a crucial step in the operation with regard to haemostasis. Failure to free the bladder adequately can result in the stapler damaging the bladder or ureter, or in incompletely securing the uterine artery pedicle. Visual clarity, and therefore haemostasis at this stage is of vital importance. This dissection requires the judicious use of laparoscopic scissors armed with monopolar coagulation diathermy, otherwise bleeding from the valveless paravesical venous plexus may ensue. Meticulous haemostasis must be maintained throughout the dissection; loss of control of even very small vessels invariably leads to diffuse haematoma formation in the loose areolar tissue of the uterovesical pouch, making visualisation difficult or impossible. Each 'bite' of tissue divided with the scissors must be checked for haemostasis before proceeding, as haematoma formation will mask any bleeding vessels and make it difficult to identify the leakage point.

Once the vaginal vault has been closed, the abdominal cavity may be reinsufflated, peritoneal toilet carried out, then a final check for haemostasis made without positive intra-abdominal pressure using the C-shaped abdominal wall retractor already described.

As the deep fascia probably never fully regains its strength after division, it is important to keep the number of laparoscopic puncture sites to a minimum. It is important that a cannula which is inadvertently withdrawn from the peritoneal cavity should be replaced in a formal manner, i.e. with the trochar fully engaged, and under direct laparoscopic vision. The initial breach in the peritoneum should be carefully negotiated, to avoid further unnecessary trauma to the peritoneum, which may occasionally be associated with brisk bleeding if a peritoneal vessel is disrupted. The 'temptation' to merely force a partially withdrawn cannula back into the peritoneal cavity (often when the tip lies within the abdominal wall, but outside the peritoneum) to save time, should be resisted. In addition to the possibility of peritoneal tears and haemorrhage, the sudden 'giving way' of the previously intact peritoneum may result in injury to abdominal viscera as the cannula is abruptly pushed into the cavity with considerable force. Herniation of gut or omentum into the incisions requiring further surgical intervention is possible, so incisions should be made as small as possible. Some authorities recommend formal closure of all entry points above

5 mm in diameter to preclude the possibility of hernia-formation. We have not so far found this necessary.

Introduction of the trochar/cannulae into the lower quadrants of the abdomen may result in damage to the inferior epigastric vessels and their branches. This may result in severe bruising of the anterior abdominal wall, which may 'track' around the lateral wall and extend to the thighs (Fig. 7.1). Abdominal wall haematomata or (rarely) significant intra-abdominal haemorrhage may also occur. These vessels may be visualised directly through the laparoscope according to some authors (Reich 1989), or in the thin patient by transillumination of the anterior abdominal wall, and thereby avoided during insertion of the lower (lateral) portals. The likelihood of this injury is increased by repeated introduction of the trochar and cannula, which may be avoided by the use of a trochar sleeve with a coarse screw profile on its outer aspect which effectively 'locks' the cannula into a fixed position in the abdominal wall (Surgigrip™, Auto Suture Company). If a vessel of significant size is damaged, the bleeding may leak from the incision or become apparent laparoscopically, usually draining along the shaft of the cannula, into the peritoneal cavity. Such bleeding is often tamponaded by the cannula; venous bleeding may often cease by the time the procedure is concluded. It is therefore important that if blood is seen to drain along the cannula inside the abdomen, unless the bleeding is obviously from a large arterial vessel, *it should not be removed,* but steps taken to control the bleeding.

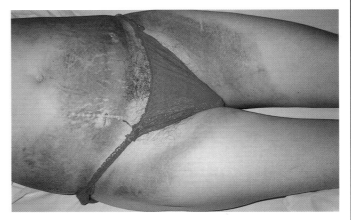

Fig. 7.1 **Extensive haematoma resulting from damage to right epigastric artery.**

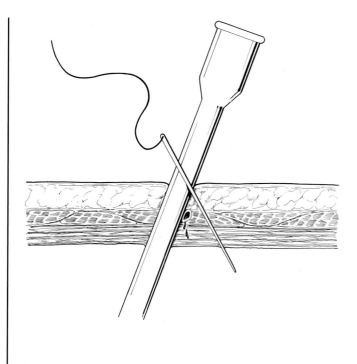

(a)

More serious bleeding may be controlled by passing a heavy gauge suture (silk number 1 is ideal) on a large straight needle through the full thickness of the abdominal wall under laparoscopic control. This is relatively easy to achieve by first passing the needle through the lateral angle of the trochar/cannula incision, lateral to the cannula, at an angle of approximately 45° such that the needle is pointing laterally. Admission to the peritoneal cavity is under direct laparoscopic vision. Once the needle has penetrated the peritoneum, it is grasped with self-locking forceps via the contralateral port, then passed through the abdominal wall again, at an angle of 45°, such that the suture encompasses at least 25 mm width of abdominal wall in the transverse plane. This time, the needle exits via the medial angle of the abdominal incision, once again at an angle of 45°, with the point facing medially. The suture is then tightly knotted on one side of the trochar. Since the injured blood vessel will almost invariably run in the 'up–down' direction, this single suture is almost always successful in arresting bleeding (Fig. 7.2). If this fails, then the artery may (rarely) need to be dissected out and ligated under direct vision.

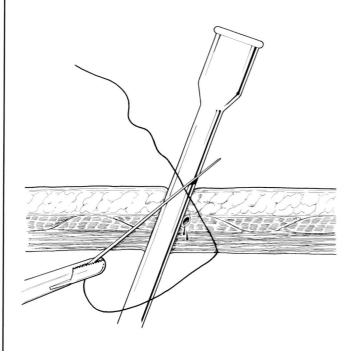

(b)

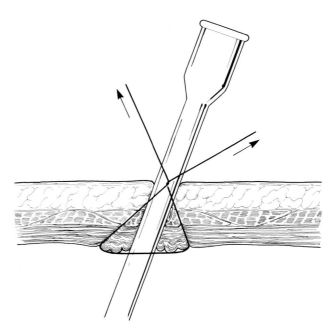

(c)

Fig. 7.2 **Endoscopic method of controlling haemorrhage from traumatised abdominal wall blood vessel.**

URETERIC INJURY

Ureteric injury may cause considerable suffering when it occurs and, needless to say, must be assiduously avoided. During 'open' abdominal hysterectomy, the differential movement of the bladder and ureters caudally and traction on the uterus cranially usually ensures that the urinary tract is clear of the operative field. At laparoscopic hysterectomy, the same degree of separation between the uterine artery and the ureter is difficult to achieve. The ureter may therefore be trapped by the stapler when used to secure and divide the uterine arteries unless care is exercised.

This injury may be avoided by several means. The ureter may be identified at the pelvic brim, dissected out and visualised, although devascularisation and consequent necrosis is a risk (cf. Wertheim's hysterectomy). Dissection and identification of the ureter is not a guarantee that ureteric injury will not occur, however (Woodland 1992). Ureteric catheterisation with transilluminating ureteric stents (Uriglow™, Rocket of London Ltd) allows identification at the time of operation and is routinely employed by the author at the present time. A high-intensity cold light source is used to illuminate the ureters, which are then easily visible as a series of glowing dots. The disadvantages of this manoeuvre are that the skill of ureteric catheterisation must be acquired and the added cost of the stents.

If ureteric injury is diagnosed peroperatively, it may be repaired as a primary procedure. Intravenous injection of indigo carmine dye has been used to locate lacerations of the ureter and either open or laparoscopic repair (Nezhat & Nezhat 1992) carried out. When there is delayed diagnosis of urinary tract damage, management is usually deemed to be within the province of the urologist. The diagnosis under these circumstances follows symptoms of urinary leakage if a fistula has developed (incontinence in the case of uretero–vaginal lesions, or peritonitis if urine leaks into the abdominal cavity), or loin/ureteric pain where there is significant obstruction to renal outflow.

BLADDER INJURY

The bladder is mainly vulnerable to injury at two stages during laparoscopic hysterectomy: firstly, when the peritoneum of the uterovesical pouch is divided and the bladder dissected free from the anterior surface of the uterus and cervix; and, secondly, when the uterine artery pedicle is stapled laparoscopically, if the bladder has not been adequately displaced downward. Since the bladder dissection is usually carried out using monopolar diathermy-armed scissors and blunt development of the tissue plane, it may be torn or thermally injured by diathermy. The latter may be especially difficult to identify, since subsequent tissue necrosis may occur only after 24 or more hours have elapsed. Moreover, the zone of necrosis around a diathermy injury may be several millimetres beyond that which is immediately apparent (Indman & Soderstrom 1990). Placing the peritoneum and extravesical tissue 'on stretch' with non-locking laparoscopic forceps to facilitate inspection of the operative field, and dissecting close to the uterine surface, will minimise the risk of injury. This step of the operation is potentially very bloody if the tissue plane is not correctly identified, resulting in poor visualisation and thus increasing the likelihood of inappropriate tissue dissection with consequent bladder injury. This dissection is more difficult if the bladder is adherent to the uterus following previous surgery.

Bladder injury identified immediately usually presents little difficulty, provided the site of the injury is not close to the ureterovesical junctions and the lesion is clearly defined. A tear in the bladder wall may be sutured in layers either laparoscopically or vaginally, depending upon where the lesion is sited, and the bladder continuously drained for at least 10 days. Urological assistance may of course be required.

URINARY TRACT INFECTION

Bladder catheterisation, pelvic surgery and reflex retention of urine because of pain all predispose to lower urinary tract infection, which is consequently a potential complication of almost all gynaecological surgery. However, ureteric catheterisation carries the additional risk of ascending infection and possible pyelonephritis. Meticulous aseptic technique and prophylactic antibiotics reduce the risk of this complication. It is important to note that ureteric catheterisation may often slightly traumatise the transitional epithelium of the ureter; transient light macroscopic haematuria is occasionally noted and in the absence of other signs and symptoms should not alarm the surgeon.

BOWEL INJURY

The steep Trendelenburg position used for laparoscopic surgery usually causes the bowel to 'pool' in the upper abdomen, leaving a clear operative field. Adhesions of the sigmoid colon and small bowel in the pelvis may require division prior to definitive surgery to ensure that the risk of bowel damage is minimised. Lacerations, crush and thermal injuries have all been described and unless immediately recognised may result in peritonitis and life-threatening illness.

Damage to bowel must *always* be treated in the conventional way, with the help of a general surgeon, in the opinion of the author. At the present time, there can be little or no place for attempts at endoscopic repair of bowel-related complications. Such attempts have led to disaster. Needle stick injuries of less than 2 mm with no observable leakage may be safely treated conservatively (Berci & Cuschieri 1986). All larger injuries are serious and require surgical intervention. Endoscopic instruments must only be used when the active end is within the field of vision, and the diathermy generator *always* deactivated when not required.

There is little question that the best way of dealing with complications of any surgery is prevention; the case for laparoscopic hysterectomy is no different. Proper patient selection is mandatory, and certainly the surgeon embarking upon advanced laparoscopic surgical techniques must be highly selective; obese patients and those who have undergone previous abdominal surgery should be avoided in the first instance. The surgeon should have made every effort to gain as much training and supervised experience as possible – ideally at first with one of the widely available bench-top training devices with video facilities (Pelvi-trainer or similar). Properly organised, preferably 'hands-on' training courses are ideal; indeed, there is no substitute at all for operating at the side of an experienced laparoscopic surgeon to obtain a true 'feel' for the techniques. Remote viewing, video recordings and so on are very poor substitutes for traditional surgical training in the 'apprentice tradition', but for those surgeons already in senior positions, the type of teaching course mentioned is invaluable.

The equipment must be appropriate, in good working order and familiar to the operator. The latter should have a good working knowledge of the equipment he is using; what it is, and is not, capable of. He should be thoroughly familiar with the application of all modes of haemostasis control at his disposal and, above all, know when to quit. Laparoscopic procedures taking several hours are rarely justified, and never when the prolonged duration is due to loss of haemostasis that proves resistant to the usual methods of control. The mark of the good laparoscopic surgeon is infinite patience, but infinite humility as well.

8

CLINICAL EXPERIENCE WITH LAPAROSCOPIC HYSTERECTOMY AND OOPHORECTOMY

Laparoscopic hysterectomy

Prospective randomised trial of laparoscopic versus 'open' hysterectomy and bilateral salpingo-oophorectomy

Current series: results and complications

Laparoscopic oophorectomy

LAPAROSCOPIC HYSTERECTOMY

Presented here are essentially two studies: firstly, a prospective, randomised trial of laparoscopic versus 'open' total hysterectomy and bilateral salpingo-oophorectomy (Phipps et al 1992), and, secondly, an up-to-date review of the series of cases dealt with in this Unit.

PROSPECTIVE, RANDOMISED TRIAL OF LAPAROSCOPIC VERSUS 'OPEN' TOTAL HYSTERECTOMY AND BILATERAL SALPINGO-OOPHORECTOMY

53 patients underwent either laparoscopic hysterectomy and bilateral salpingo-oophorectomy (24 patients) or open total abdominal hysterectomy and bilateral salpingo-oophorectomy via a traditional transverse suprapubic incision (29 patients).

In this study we compared the laparoscopic technique with its open counterpart with respect to operative time, postoperative analgesia requirements, length of stay in hospital, convalescence time and cost. Patients were admitted to the trial if hysterectomy and bilateral oophorectomy were indicated because of menorrhagia (including dysfunctional uterine bleeding (DUB) and fibroids of 8 weeks' gestational size or less), where oophorectomy was included because of cyclic pelvic pain, severe premenstrual syndrome (PMS) or because of the patient's wishes in those given the option over the age of 45. Patients with stage I endometrial carcinoma, diagnosed by hysteroscopy and endo-metrial biopsy, were also admitted. Chest X-ray and liver function tests were normal. Patients were randomly assigned to undergo either operation. No patient had undergone previous gynaecological surgery.

There were no significant differences between groups of patients with respect to indication for surgery, uterine size, age or parity (Tables 8.1 and 8.2). There were no operative or postoperative complications. In the three patients with endometrial carcinoma, there was no evidence of extrauterine spread of disease and histological examination revealed tumours confined to the endometrial cavity.

Table 8.1 **Patient characteristics**

	Laparoscopic surgery (n = 24)	Open surgery (n = 29)
Uterine size normal	18 (75.0%)	25 (86.2%)
≤ 6 weeks	3 (12.5%)	2 (6.9%)
≤ 8 weeks	3 (12.5%)	2 (6.9%)
Mean age (range)	41 (32–51)	39 (30–50)
Mean parity (range)	1.5 (0–5)	2.0 (0–4)

Table 8.2 **Indications for surgery**

	Laparoscopic surgery (n = 24)	Open surgery (n = 29)
DUB/fibroids+ PMS	10 (41.7%)	10 (34.5%)
DUB/fibroids + patient elected for BSO	7 (29.2%)	10 (34.5%)
Pelvic pain	6 (25.0%)	7 (24.1%)
Stage I endometrial carcinoma	1 (4.2%)	2 (6.9%)

Operative time was significantly longer in the laparoscopic group: mean 65 min (range 44–110 min), laparotomy 30 min (range 18–40 min, $p = < 0.001$), but there was a marked learning curve. The first laparoscopic operation took 1 h 50 min to complete, whereas the last five have all taken approximately 1 h. The average cost of the laparoscopic procedure was approximately ten times that of the open operation (cost of Multifire Endo GIA™ disposable stapler, three extra staple cartridges, two disposable 12 mm trochar and cannulae, a vacuum drain and two sutures approximately £500.00; cost of eight sutures for open procedure approximately £50.00).

The advantages in terms of patient comfort, time taken to return to work and bed occupancy were clear. On average, patients in the laparoscopic group required 1.5 (range 0–3) 10 mg doses of intramuscular morphine compared to 4.5 (range 3–10) doses in the laparotomy group ($p = < 0.001$) after surgery.

Median stay in hospital after laparoscopic surgery was significantly shorter compared to open surgery: 48 h

(range 36–60 h) compared to 6 d (range 5–7 d, $p = < 0.001$). Patients returned to work after laparoscopic surgery after 2–4 weeks (median 2 weeks), whereas after open surgery they required 5–7 weeks' convalescence (median 6 weeks, $p = < 0.001$).

CURRENT SERIES: LAPAROSCOPIC HYSTERECTOMY WITH AND WITHOUT BILATERAL SALPINGO-OOPHORECTOMY: RESULTS AND COMPLICATIONS

Indications for laparoscopic hysterectomy with and without BSO are shown in Table 8.3. Patients with dysfunctional uterine bleeding had declined endometrial ablation (either transcervical resection or radiofrequency endometrial ablation – RaFEA), usually because absolute amenorrhoea could not be guaranteed. Patients with fibroids had a uterine size of 12 weeks' gestation or less. Patients with stage I endometrial carcinoma had previously undergone diagnostic hysteroscopy and confirmative endometrial biopsy.

Table 8.3 **Current series: indications for surgery**

LH with BSO (n = 145)	
DUB with cyclic pelvic pain	48/145 (33.1%)
DUB with PMS	23/145 (15.9%)
Fibroids/menorrhagia with pelvic pain*	19/145 (13.1%)
Fibroids/menorrhagia with PMS *	11/145 (7.6%)
Age >45; patient elected for BSO	42/145 (29.1%)
Stage I endometrial carcinoma	2/145 (1.4%)
LH alone (n = 78)	
Clinical indication for simple hysterectomy plus poor vaginal access ± poor descent	70/78 (88.6%)
Adhesions/endometriosis	8/78 (10.3%)

* Uterus of 12 weeks' gestation size or less

Operative time for procedures including the uterine artery dissection laparoscopically was 60–120 min (mean 78 min), and for those where the uterine artery was included in the vaginal dissection was 50–100 min (mean 65 min). Placement of transilluminating ureteric stents did not add significantly to the operative time because this was achieved simultaneously with the placing of the abdominal trochar/cannulae.

The median time in hospital following surgery is 48 h (range 36 h–8 d). Patients are followed up at two and twelve weeks postoperatively. The median convalescence time is 3 weeks before returning to normal activity (range 1–8 weeks).

There were four cases of primary haemorrhage, all of which required laparotomy and resuturing of the uterine artery. In all cases patients were noticed to be losing excessive amounts of blood into their drain (>200 ml of blood or blood mixed with saline). All four required blood transfusion (2–6 units). In each case, the reason for loss of haemostasis was identical. A small area had been inadvertently left unsecured between the inferior margin of the laparoscopic staple line and the top of the vaginal dissection. Small branches of the uterine artery were therefore unsecured (see Ch. 7).

The patient who suffered ureteric injury presented 10 days postoperatively complaining of severe right-sided loin pain and fever. On examination, she was tender in the right costophrenic angle and had a temperature of 37.8°C. An emergency intravenous urogram (IVU) showed a normally functioning kidney and ureter on the left side, but an enlarged poorly functioning kidney and distended ureter on the right. There was evidence of leakage of urine from the distal end of the occluded ureter. Although the ureteric shadow could be seen to continue past the staple line, there was evidence of occlusion just proximal to the ureterovesical junction. A laparotomy was performed, with urological help, and the right ureter re-implanted without difficulty or complication. The distal 15 mm of ureter had become acutely kinked and had undergone necrosis as a result of a vaginal suture which had been placed high up and laterally to secure some bleeding from an unsecured gap between the laparoscopic and vaginal dissections. Ureteric stents had not been prophylactically used in this case. Indirectly, therefore, this complication was essentially due to the same fault as the cases of haemorrhage. At 6 weeks' follow-up, the patient was well and asymptomatic, and a repeat IVU showed a normally functioning urinary tract.

One patient developed pelvic abscess after surgery, but had not received prophylactic antibiotics. The operation was uncomplicated, and lasted 60 min. She was discharged home after 48 h, but returned 3 days later complaining of abdominal pain. On examination, there was marked peritonism and a palpable mass at the vaginal vault. In view of the clinical signs suggestive of general peritonitis, a laparotomy was performed. This revealed no abnormality at the operative site, but multiple abscesses scattered around the peritoneal cavity. The sigmoid colon and left ovary were involved in a large abscess, and general surgical assistance was obtained. The sigmoid colon was not breached, but was very friable, and a defunctioning colostomy was performed with drainage of the abscess. There was no evidence of previous postoperative haemorrhage. The patient recovered well, and was discharged home after 10 days. 2 months later the colostomy was reversed, and she is now well and asymptomatic.

The mechanism of this complication is unclear; there was no evidence to suggest that a predisposing haematoma following surgery had developed. We presume that there was a pre-existing subclinical salpingitis at the time of surgery. Cultures taken at the time of laparotomy were sterile. A full regime of antibiotic prophylaxis is now given to all patients; no further infective complications have been encountered.

LAPAROSCOPIC OOPHORECTOMY

At the time of writing, 38 laparoscopic oophorectomies have been performed in this unit, using the technique described in this manual. The indication for surgery was adjuvant treatment of breast cancer in all but two cases (36/38, 94.7%). The remaining two patients (5.3%) suffered intractable cyclic pelvic pain having previously undergone hysterectomy for a benign indication. No major complications have been encountered, although one patient drained 150 ml blood of unknown origin into the vacuum drain. She made an otherwise uneventful recovery. The mean operating time was 21 min (range 18–35 min), and the median postoperative hospital stay was 24 h (range 24–72 h). Convalescence time was 1–2 weeks (median 1 week).

It seems likely that as long as general surgeons are again convinced of the value of oophorectomy as an adjuvant therapy for breast cancer, this will be an operation much in demand. Certainly, the same criticisms levelled against laparoscopic hysterectomy, that in many cases a more straightforward and cheaper route exists (vaginal hysterectomy), cannot be put forward against oophorectomy. The alternative to a quick and relatively atraumatic laparoscopic excision is, in all cases, a laparotomy with all the attendant problems. For those who remain unconvinced of the value of laparoscopic hysterectomy, laparoscopic oophorectomy should not be considered in the same light at all.

9

MINIMALLY INVASIVE SURGERY:
a primary health care perspective

P. J. Lefley

The introduction of minimally invasive surgery across a whole variety of disciplines brings both opportunities and problems for the family doctor. At a time when many specialties are confessing to their difficulties in keeping up with the latest advances in their field, the generalist is even more hard pressed to stay abreast with the ever-increasing rate of progress across a broad front. An incident which occurred locally illustrates the point. A GP was asked to see a woman with abdominal pain, bleeding and a positive pregnancy test. On bimanual examination she was tender in the right fornix. The practitioner admitted her to hospital with a provisional diagnosis of ectopic pregnancy. 2 days later, he was surprised to see her in morning surgery. Unsure of whether his original diagnosis had been correct (despite her assurances that it was), he asked her to lie on the examination couch so that he could see the scars from her surgery himself. Confronted with three small puncture wounds and a patient who had been discharged from hospital barely 24 h after admission, he told her that she could not possibly have had an ectopic pregnancy, and that the laparoscopy must have confirmed that. Unfortunately the doctor was unaware that tubal pregnancies can be removed laparoscopically, and that the procedure had recently been introduced at his local hospital. Equally unfortunate was the fact that a discharge summary had not reached him before the patient had.

This story illustrates the problems inherent in being unaware of advances in surgical techniques. Needless to say, the confidence of the patient was not enhanced by her doctor appearing ignorant of the operation, although in this case she received treatment which was both timely and appropriate. What if the practitioner had a choice of two or three local hospitals to refer to, where minimally invasive surgery might or might not be available? Then his lack of knowledge of new procedures would put his patient at a significant disadvantage. This is even more so where elective procedures such as hysterectomy and oophorectomy are concerned. The clear message is that a close liaison between primary health care practitioners and specialist provider units must be forged. This will provide information for the GP on the range of services provided, and what both he and the patient may expect from them. Patients locally are provided with an information sheet which gives them an outline of their operation and answers the most frequently asked questions. This is good practice, and a copy of these information sheets will answer a similar number of questions which the GP may have:

THROUGH THE KEYHOLE

A PATIENT'S GUIDE TO ENDOSCOPIC GYNAECOLOGICAL SURGERY

What is endoscopic surgery?

Endoscopic surgery means that the surgical procedure is carried out through very small incisions in the abdomen or through the neck of the womb (the *cervix*). The advantage of this type of approach is that no large cut has to be made in the abdomen, which means that recovery is much faster, and of course there is no large scar left after the operation. Surgery is carried out using special telescopes called endoscopes, which are inserted either through the umbilicus ('belly button') for laparoscopic surgery inside the abdomen, or through the cervix (*hysteroscopic surgery*) for operating inside the womb. The endoscope is then attached to a miniature colour video camera which in turn transmits the picture to a video monitor screen. If the operation is inside the abdomen, two more small punctures in the abdominal wall lower down (just on the line of the pubic hair) are necessary to insert very long, narrow instruments which are used to perform the surgery. The surgeon then watches the operation on the video screen. It is important to appreciate that, for technical reasons, it may be necessary to revert to a traditional 'open' operation during the course of any keyhole surgery. This is very unusual, but may occasionally be required.

Can all operations be performed this way?

No. In some cases, for example in women with very large uterine fibroids, the womb is too large to be removed safely using these 'keyhole' techniques and a more traditional operation must be carried out through a larger incision. In other cases, it may be essential to take samples from other parts of the abdomen, which sometimes means that a traditional surgical incision must be made.

What operations can be performed?

In gynaecology, most of the procedures traditionally performed through 'open' surgery may now be performed using these new endoscopic techniques. The most often performed 'keyhole' procedures are:

Laparoscopic hysterectomy

This is the removal of the whole womb, including the cervix, using keyhole techniques. The advantage over traditional hysterectomy is that there is no large scar, the time in hospital is much less (usually only 2–3 days), and the recovery period is much shorter (2–3 weeks). Unlike endometrial ablation, a guarantee may be made that absolutely no more periods will occur, but it is a bigger operation than endometrial ablation (although not as traumatic, of course, as a traditional hysterectomy). If there is any reason to remove the ovaries (such as cysts), then this may be done at the same time. You should discuss this matter with your gynaecologist before the operation.

Laparoscopic oophorectomy

This means the removal of both ovaries using keyhole surgery and may usually be done with only a single overnight stay in hospital. The womb is not affected. This operation is sometimes necessary for women with breast trouble, or those with ovarian cysts, and avoids the trauma of major surgery.

   Whichever operation is recommended to you, you should consider it very carefully and discuss the various options with your gynaecologist.

The following is an example of the information sheet routinely given to patients after undergoing minimally invasive gynaecological surgery, before discharge from hospital. Subsequent calls to the GP are thereby kept to a minimum.

AFTER MINIMALLY INVASIVE GYNAECOLOGICAL SURGERY

What to expect after gynaecological minimally invasive or 'keyhole' surgery depends upon which operation you have undergone. There are, however, general principles to bear in mind when recovering from such an operation. This information sheet will explain these, and then go on to explain about specific individual operations.

First and foremost, it is important that you (and your family!) remember that, while you may have either no scars at all or very small scars, nevertheless, you have undergone major surgery – it's just that you can't see the scars because they are inside. It is therefore important that you get plenty of rest for 1–3 weeks after surgery (depending upon which operation has been carried out), otherwise you will feel very tired most of the day. This is because your body is healing and therefore requires considerably more energy than usual. If antibiotics are given to you, it is *most* important that you take them to guard you against infection. Depending upon the operation you have had, you may or may not need them – you will be advised.

LAPAROSCOPIC HYSTERECTOMY AND/OR OOPHORECTOMY

This is removal of the womb (hysterectomy) with or without removal of the ovaries (oophorectomy). Although you cannot see very much on the outside, remember that this is a major operation. After surgery, you may need 2–4 weeks away from work or normal duties. Some irregular vaginal bleeding and discharge (often with small pieces of stitch in it) is quite normal and this should not alarm you. This is caused by healing of the vault (top) of the vagina, where the womb has been removed. You should not have intercourse or use tampons for 3 weeks after surgery. You will be given 10 days' supply of antibiotics – it is *essential* that you take the full course.

If your operation has included surgery for incontinence of urine, you may well find that passing water is a bit strange for several months. This is because the bladder is in a completely new position and your body has to get used to it.

Whichever operation you have undergone it is important to avoid sexual intercourse for at least 3 weeks, unless you have been told to the contrary.

Depending upon which operation you have had, you will be seen in the outpatient clinic between 2 weeks and 3 months after surgery.

To supplement these written guidelines, postgraduate meetings between the primary health care team and specialist unit are a useful adjunct. The whole field of minimally invasive surgery lends itself to high quality audiovisual presentations, and these provide a fascinating insight for the uninitiated into the nuts and bolts of endoscopic surgery.

The final aim of all links between primary care physicians and specialists is to provide a so-called 'seamless service' for the patient. In times past it has been all too common for 'the right hand not to know what the left is doing' (to use an English colloquialism) – in other words, incoordination between referring GP and specialist. The primary health care doctor is reliant upon his specialist colleagues' skill and expertise. However, particularly in light of the Health Service reforms in the UK, the specialist is increasingly dependent on the GP for patient referrals. This trend is gaining momentum in the US, where patients now frequently belong to medical organisations whose insurance companies insist on the so-called 'gate-keeping' activity of a primary health care physician before accepting liability for paying the specialist's fees. Close cooperation makes plain sense when considering the single most important factor in the equation: the patient's interests. Close cooperation also makes sense for the specialist who wishes to maximise his clinical activity.

It is quite common for patients to visit their family doctor for an explanation of what has been done to them while they were in hospital, despite all the efforts of the specialist and his hospital staff. In areas where there has been a total breakdown of communication between the hospital and general practice, I would support the creation of a national prize for the generalist who is best able to explain to a patient an operation which he has never heard of, let alone understood. Before gynaecologists smile too broadly, a second prize might be given for the best dissertation on 'how depressive illness can lead to pelvic evisceration'(!)

So...having been armed with the knowledge of what operations are technically possible and what is involved, what are the benefits for patients which will persuade their GP to refer them for this type of surgery? From the patients' perspective, the absence of a large scar is obviously an attractive proposition. This, coupled with a reduction in general surgical trauma, has enabled hospital stays in many cases to be reduced dramatically. The reduced morbidity evidenced by shortened hospital stays is also reflected in the community. Patients recuperate faster and can return to work earlier. Hopefully, the days when a hysterectomy is seen as an automatic entitlement to 3 months' sick leave are numbered. Indeed, some patients are rather taken aback when the advice they are given on returning to work clashes with what has become folklore handed down by generations of women who have 'had it all taken away'. It is therefore an occasional paradox that the assurance that a patient may return to work in 2–3 weeks rather than 12 is not always well received.

A further factor influencing referral is pressure exerted by patients themselves to have a particular type of treatment. Morbid enthusiasm generated by the media for more and more lurid details of medicine's innermost secrets brings in its trail a cult of dedicated followers determined to be the recipients of the perceived benefits of the latest development. Sometimes these requests are reasonable, sometimes not. Forewarned is forearmed. It is important for the generalist to be in a position of knowledge so that a sound judgement may be made on whether or not a particular request is reasonable. Once again, a sound relationship between patient, generalist and specialist will ensure appropriate referrals such that the consumers of health care receive treatment which is best suited to their needs.

Once patients have returned to the community from hospital, the GP may be called to see them for a variety of reasons. Because of the paucity of evidence of surgical trauma externally, he should be mindful that internally major surgery may have been undertaken. Consequently, the complications of major surgery are possible and nearly all of these will require the patient to be seen by the specialist unit. While a superficial wound infection can be treated in the community, any suggestion of intra-abdominal abnormality will require admission. The GP must be aware of the possible complications attendant upon minimally invasive surgery, including secondary haemorrhage and ureteric injury. Loin pain or incontinence should be treated as evidence of ureteric or bladder damage until proven otherwise. In general, however, it is hoped that as specialist units gain more experience the incidence of postoperative complications should become less common than those associated with open surgery. This is especially true for nosocomial infections and thromboembolic disease, because of the reduced time in hospital after surgery.

Continuing the theme of close cooperation between hospitals and general practice, specialists should be candid with regard to surgical complications and clear about their rationale for declining to operate laparoscopically on particular patients. The specialist should make the results of his clinical audit openly available to the referring generalist. In the past, such statistics were considered 'secret' and the exclusion of unsuitable patients from a particular mode of treatment was seen as a kind of weakness or admission of a less than perfect technique. Such attitudes are no longer acceptable. Open discussion of complication risks between all three parties prior to surgery can lead to a much better outcome if things do go awry.

Specialists may or may not be aware that a remarkable 'bush telegraph' operates amongst GPs, and I am advised by my American generalist colleagues that this is certainly also the case in the US. If a ureter has been divided, it is better that the referring doctor is made aware of it first through conventional channels, without lurid and misinformed embellishments. It is also a fact that despite any number of statistics, if a major complication does occur, then for the patient (and often the referring doctor) it has occurred in a series of one. All operations naturally carry a complication rate; only open discussion of these will silence the 'bush telegraph'. Specialists might like to ponder Deming's attitude, which applies itself broadly to this: satisfied customers (patients and referring doctors) are not good enough – they have to become 'walking advertisements' for the service (Walton 1986).

Armed with information about availability, an outline content of the operation and morbidity statistics, a further part of the equation which is becoming more prominent in the decision to refer patients for surgery is cost. The 'fund-holding initiative' in the United Kingdom has placed GPs in a position of control of their budgets for elective surgery and outpatient appointments – much along the lines of the US system. The ability to switch savings from this budget to other areas of practice is making fund-holding practices pay particular attention to treatment costs. As already mentioned, in the United States, concern over the escalation of health care cost has led to an increase in the number of primary care physicians providing a 'gate-keeper service' and it seems likely that this trend will continue. Indeed, the main focus in the Western world for the foreseeable future will be on containing medical costs.

Minimally invasive surgery is being introduced at a propitious time with relation to these pressures. Although operative costs are higher, considerable savings are possible due to early discharge, short convalescence time and early return to work. This results in the overall cost for a procedure falling and hence the referring doctor, if he has budgetary restraints, is offered a further reason for choosing to refer his patient for minimally invasive surgery in preference to the 'open' option. In addition to cost reduction, the productivity of provider units should be able to increase because of a downward pressure on bed occupancy. This will result in shorter waiting lists and a reduced number of inpatient beds.

I began this chapter by saying that minimally invasive surgery offers both opportunities and potential problems for the family doctor, and I have briefly outlined these. The ultimate goal must be to maximise the opportunities and eliminate the problems. Specialists will have their own strategies to tackle this equation; generalists will inevitably develop theirs, based on their perception of the specialist's performance in dealing with both themselves and their patients. The key to success is a close working relationship between specialist and generalist, which must include the free exchange of information. When the relationship is at its best, patients will flow smoothly from the community to hospital to receive sophisticated treatment, then back to the community. This is the generalist's aim, and only the specialist can help him realise it. The Holy Grail of all medical care must be continuous improvement; there is no question that these gynaecological minimally invasive procedures are a very significant step forward. If specialist and generalist work closely together, continuous improvement will be assured.

REFERENCES

Arthure H 1970 Laparoscopy hazards. Brit Med J 4: 492

Barker P, Langton J A, Murphy P J, Rowbotham D J 1992 Regurgitation of gastric contents during general anaesthesia using the laryngeal mask airway. Brit J Anaes 69: 314–315

Barnett R, Gallant B, Fossey S, Finegan B 1992 A comparison between face-mask, laryngeal mask and endotracheal intubation. Can J Anaes 395 (5): 151

Berci G, Cuschieri A 1986 Practical laparoscopy. Blackwell, London, p 172

Bruhat M A, Mage G, Chapron C, Pouly J L, Canis M, Wattiez A 1991 Present day endoscopic surgery in gynaecology. Eur J Obstet Gynecol Reprod Biol 41 (1): 4–13

Chamberlain G, Brown J 1978 Gynaecological laparoscopy; report of the Working Party of the Confidential Enquiry Into Gynaecological Laparoscopy. Royal College of Obstetricians and Gynaecologists, London

Cooney C M, Lyons J B, Hennigan A, Blunnie W P, Moriarty D C 1992 Ventilatory function following laparoscopic cholecystectomy. Can J Anaes 395 (5): A54

Daly J W, Higgins K A 1988 Injury to the ureter during gynecologic surgical procedures. Surg Gynecol Obstet 167: 19–22

Dicker R C, Greenspan J R, Strauss L T 1982 Complications of abdominal and vaginal hysterectomy among women of reproductive age in the United States. Am J Obstet Gynecol 144: 841–848

Duff P, Park R C 1980 Antibiotic prophylaxis in vaginal hysterectomy: a review. Obstet Gynecol 55: 1935

Gabbot D A, Dunkley A B, Roberts F L 1992 Carbon dioxide pneumothorax occurring during laparoscopic cholecystectomy. Anaesthesia 47: 587

Garry R 1992 Laparoscopic alternatives to laparotomy: a new approach to gynaecological surgery. Brit J Obstet Gynaecol 99 (8): 629–632

Hahn G M 1982 Hyperthermia and cancer. Springer-Verlag, New York, pp 4–32

Hester J B, Heath M L 1977. Pulmonary acid aspiration syndrome: should prophylaxis be routine? Brit J Anaes 49: 595–599

Indman P D, Soderstrom R M 1990 Depth of endometrial coagulation with the urologic resectoscope. J Reprod Med 35 (6): 633–635

Johns A 1991 Laparoscopic oophorectomy/oophorocystectomy. Clin Obstet Gynecol 34 (2): 460–466

Knas G B 1991 Pneumopericardium associated with laparoscopy. Am J Clin Anes 3: 56

Magos A L, Broadbent J A, Amso N N 1991 Laparoscopically assisted vaginal hysterectomy (letter). Lancet 338: 1091–1092

Maher P J, Hill D J 1991 Video assisted laparoscopic vaginal hysterectomy (letter). Med J Aust 154 (6): 427

Minelli L, Angiolillo M, Caione C, Palmara V 1991 Laparoscopically assisted vaginal hysterectomy. Endoscopy 23 (2): 64–66

Nezhat C, Nezhat F 1992 Laparoscopic repair of ureter resected during operative laparoscopy. Obstet Gynecol 80: 543–544

Nezhat F, Nezhat C, Silfsen S L 1991 Videolaseroscopy for oophorectomy. Am J Obstet Gynecol 165 (5;1): 1323–1330

Nezhat F, Nezhat C, Gordon S, Wilkins E 1992 Laparoscopic versus abdominal hysterectomy. J Reprod Med 37 (3): 247–250

Phipps J H, Tyrrell N J 1992 Transilluminating ureteric stents for preventing operative ureteric damage. Brit J Obstet Gynaecol 99: 81

Phipps J H, John M, Nayak S 1992 Laparoscopically-assisted vaginal hysterectomy and bilateral salpingoophorectomy versus open abdominal hysterectomy and bilateral salpingoophorectomy. Brit J Obstet Gynaecol (in press)

Polk B F, Shapiro M, Goldstein P 1980 Randomized clinical trial of perioperative cephazolin in preventing infection after hysterectomy. Lancet i: 437

Reich H 1989a New techniques in advanced laparoscopic surgery. Baill Clin Obstet Gynaecol 3 (3): 655–681

Reich H 1989b Laparoscopic oophorectomy without ligature or morcellation. Contemp Obstet Gynecol 9: 34–46

Reich H, DeCapria J, McGlynn F 1989 Laparoscopic hysterectomy. J Gynecol Surg 1 (5): 213

Reich H, McGlynn F, Wilkie W 1990 Laparoscopic management of stage I ovarian cancer. A case report. J Reprod Med 35 (6): 1285–1290

Reid C W, Martineau R J, Hull K A, Miller D R 1992 Haemodynamic consequences of abdominal insufflation with carbon dioxide during laparoscopic cholecystectomy. Can J Anaes 395 (5): A132

Salzman E W, Hirsh J 1982 Prevention of venous thromboembolism. In: Colman R W, Hirsh J, Marden V, Salzman E W (eds) Hemostasis and thrombosis: basic principles and clinical practice. Lippincott, New York, p 986

Scrimgeour J B, Ng K B, Gaudoin M R 1991 Laparoscopy in vaginal hysterectomy (letter). Lancet 338: 1465–1466

Sharp F, Jordan J A 1987 Gynaecological laser surgery. Perinatology Press, New York, p 266

Stirrat G M, Dwyer N, Browning J 1990 Planned trial of transcervical resection of the endometrium versus hysterectomy. Br J Obstet Gynaecol 97 (5): 459

Taylor E, Feinstein R, White P F, Soper N 1992 Anaesthesia for laparoscopic cholecystectomy; is nitrous oxide contraindicated? Anesthesiology 76: 541–543

Tiret L, Desmonts J M, Hatton F, Vourch G 1986 Complications associated with anaesthesia – a prospective survey in France. Can Anaes Soc J 33 (3): 336–344

Walton M 1986 The Deming management method. Mercury Business Books, London, pp 25–49

Woodland M B 1992 Ureter injury during laparoscopy-assisted vaginal hysterectomy with the endoscopic linear stapler. Am J Obstet Gynecol 167: 756–757

INDEX

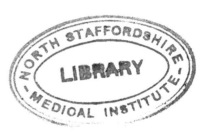